Praise for 12 Principles for Raising a Child with ADHD

"When my son got his diagnosis, I felt overwhelmed. There is so much ADHD information out there, and not all of it is helpful. I have struggled to really understand my son and how to help him—but this book has changed all that. We are finally rebuilding the connection that I thought was lost forever. Thank you, Dr. Barkley."
                    —*Krystle B., Gladstone, Australia*

"Dr. Barkley dives right into parents' most pressing questions and offers practical, science-backed guidance. This book will be at the top of my list to recommend to parents."
                    —*Stephen P. Becker, PhD, Division of Behavioral Medicine*
                    and Clinical Psychology, Cincinnati Children's Hospital
                    Medical Center

"A 'must read.' Dr. Barkley's advice about managing a household with a child with ADHD has reduced stress in every aspect of our lives. He thoughtfully emphasizes the importance of self-care, which many parents underestimate. Dr. Barkley's insights gave us a much better understanding of our child, and are thoroughly life changing!"
                    —*Jennie R., Hoboken, NJ*

"With compassion and understanding, Barkley gives you realistic, concrete approaches for the challenging process of raising a child with ADHD. The book helps you understand how your child's brain works, why they struggle, and how to help them develop the skills to be successful in life. Highly recommended!"
                    —*Kathleen Nadeau, PhD, Clinical Director,*
                    Chesapeake Center for ADHD,
                    Learning and Behavioral Health, Bethesda, Maryland

12 PRINCIPLES FOR RAISING
A CHILD WITH ADHD

Selected Works from Russell A. Barkley

For more information, visit the author's website:
www.russellbarkley.org

Taking Charge of ADHD, Fourth Edition:
The Complete, Authoritative Guide for Parents
Russell A. Barkley

Taking Charge of Adult ADHD
Russell A. Barkley with Christine M. Benton

Your Defiant Child, Second Edition:
Eight Steps to Better Behavior
Russell A. Barkley and Christine M. Benton

Your Defiant Teen, Second Edition:
10 Steps to Resolve Conflict and Rebuild Your Relationship
Russell A. Barkley and Arthur L. Robin with Christine M. Benton

12 Principles for Raising a Child with ADHD

RUSSELL A. BARKLEY, PhD

THE GUILFORD PRESS
New York   London

The information in this volume is not intended as a substitute for consultation with healthcare professionals. Each individual's health concerns should be evaluated by a qualified professional.

Purchasers of this book have permission to copy the Behavior Report Card (p. 95) and the 12 Principles for Raising a Child with ADHD (p. 176) for personal use or use with clients. These materials may be copied from the book or accessed directly from the publisher's website, but may not be stored on or distributed from intranet sites, Internet sites, or file-sharing sites, or made available for resale. No other part of this book may be reproduced, translated, stored in a retrieval system, or transmitted, in any form or by any means, electronic, mechanical, photocopying, microfilming, recording, or otherwise, without written permission from the publisher.

Printed in the United States of America

Last digit is print number: 9   8   7   6   5   4   3

Library of Congress Cataloging-in-Publication Data

Names: Barkley, Russell A., 1949– author.
Title: 12 principles for raising a child with ADHD / Russell A. Barkley, PhD.
Other titles: Twelve principles for raising a child with ADHD
Description: New York : The Guilford Press, [2021] | Includes bibliographical
    references and index.
Identifiers: LCCN 2020028893 | ISBN 9781462544448 (hardcover) | ISBN
    9781462542550 (paperback)
Subjects: LCSH: Attention-deficit-disordered-children—Family relationships. |
    Parents of attention-deficit-disordered children. | Child rearing.
Classification: LCC RJ506.H9 B366 2021 | DDC 618.92/8589—dc23
LC record available at https://lccn.loc.gov/2020028893

For my grandchildren,
the lights and loves of my life:

Claire, Will, Liam, and Craig

CONTENTS

Purchasers of this book can download and print
enlarged versions of the Behavior Report Card (p. 95)
and 12 Principles for Raising a Child with ADHD (p. 176) at
www.guilford.com/barkley27-forms for personal use or use
with clients (see copyright page for details).

AUTHOR'S NOTE

Identifying details in all of the case illustrations in this book are either thoroughly disguised to protect families' privacy or composites of real children I've known in my clinical practice.

In this book, I alternate between masculine and feminine pronouns when referring to specific individuals. I have made this choice to promote ease of reading as our language continues to evolve and not out of disrespect toward readers who identify with other personal pronouns. I sincerely hope that all will feel included.

PREFACE

Thank you for choosing to read this book. I hope it will serve as an indispensable guide as you go about the daily business of caring for and raising your child or teen with attention-deficit/hyperactivity disorder (ADHD). My goal is to introduce you to the touchstones that I've found so valuable over almost 50 years of working with parents and their children, to offer a book that you'll turn to over and over as you try to do what's best not only for a son or daughter who's dealing with ADHD but also for the rest of your family. I'm confident that by adopting the dozen principles in this book you'll have fewer and less serious difficulties raising your child, a much greater sense of competence and self-confidence as a parent, greater peace in your family, and a considerably more well-adjusted child or teen with ADHD.

If you're familiar with my best-selling book *Taking Charge of ADHD,* you may wonder why I decided to write another book for parents on this disorder. After all, the subtitle of that book is *The Complete, Authoritative Guide for Parents,* and it's now in its fourth edition. The answer is pretty simple: Parents of children with ADHD are pressed for time and for reliable solutions to everyday challenges. From the hundreds of families to whom I've provided clinical services, and from feedback on more than 800 lectures, I've learned that parents need a handful of clear guidelines that will keep them grounded in their intention to raise a happy, healthy child in spite of ADHD. Such guidelines, centered in a solid understanding of what they're dealing with, can equip them with proven practical solutions when they are struggling with the challenges of having ADHD in the family. That's what you'll find in this book.

Taking Charge of ADHD offers in-depth information on all aspects of ADHD from my own research and my weekly reviews of the latest scientific literature. This new book is based on the same up-to-date research data and clinical wisdom, but it's imbued with another dimension, one that is more directly a product of my own personal and professional evolution. As I've worked with those thousands of parents all around the world, my compassion and empathy for the people who are so devoted to their child's well-being have grown exponentially. At the same time, I've gotten a firsthand look at what it's like to care so deeply for a child with a disorder and to be determined to set that child on a course toward health, well-being, and success. Several years ago, I became the grandfather of a child on the autism spectrum, and since then I've been given the gift of actively participating in helping him overcome the challenges of autism spectrum disorder (ASD). Watching my grandson achieve daily developmental victories has been a great joy and has motivated me to try to support parents of children with ADHD in the same way that I encourage you to shepherd your own child toward the best life he or she can have.

So, I hope this book will be not just a concise practical resource but also a comfort and an inspiration. When your fifth grader suddenly remembers after dinner that he has to make a diorama to turn in tomorrow morning, I hope you'll turn to Principle 2 to renew your patience by reminding yourself that he has a disorder—and what that means to your everyday reality. When the invitation to a classmate's birthday party sends chills of terror down your spine, I'd like to think you'll turn to Principle 12 for help in anticipating the chaos and planning how your daughter can avoid disintegrating in its midst. When you throw up your hands at all the abandoned, ignored, or half-finished chores your child with ADHD has racked up, or how many house rules he's broken just this morning, I hope you'll read the section on Principle 4 and remember not to sweat the small stuff, especially when it just doesn't add up to promoting the big stuff you want for your child and your family.

You'll find these types of support and advice and a lot more in the following pages. Remember, these are *guiding* principles, meant to steer you along the path that only you can chart. Also remember that you can turn to *Taking Charge of ADHD* for details that will help you draw your map and stay on track.

HOW TO USE THIS BOOK

You can use this book as I just described—flipping to the help you desperately need at a moment when you're struggling with a particular challenge commonly presented by ADHD. You can also read the book from cover to cover and then go back to individual chapters as you need them. (And incidentally, by "you" and "parents" throughout this book I mean to include stepparents, foster parents, grandparents, and anyone else who has primary responsibility for raising a child with ADHD.)

The introductory chapter and first five principles provide a foundation for parenting a child with ADHD—understanding the keys to success (#1), remembering that your child isn't behaving "badly" because he's "bad" but because he has a developmental disorder (#2), getting into the mindset of a shepherd (#3), getting your priorities straight (#4), and becoming more mindful of your child and your interactions with him or her in each moment (#5). The other seven principles turn to more pragmatic solutions to the problems that ADHD symptoms impose on your child (and you): how to use rewards and touch versus talk to encourage desired behavior, how to compensate for your child's problems with time and memory, how to help your child get organized to succeed at school and elsewhere, how to make problem solving tangible and concrete, and how to prevent ADHD from making it hard to leave home. If you haven't read *Taking Charge of ADHD*, I recommend you first read the Introduction, where you'll get a short course in the developmental nature of ADHD and how that translates to what you see in your child's daily functioning. This understanding is critical to effectively adopting all of the 12 principles in this book. The Conclusion will be invaluable for its vision of how the 12 principles come together into effective, rewarding parenting of a child with ADHD.

I deeply appreciate the advice and assistance of Kitty Moore and Chris Benton of The Guilford Press for making this book a far better product and for bringing the book to production. And thanks as always to my friends Seymour Weingarten, Editor in Chief, and Bob Matloff, President, at Guilford for their continued support of my many books and my newsletter, rating scales, and other products over the 38 years that I have been publishing with them. Finally, I want to thank the thousands of parents of children and teens with ADHD with whom I have worked over my more than 40-year career for giving me so much insight into and advice about how best to raise a child with ADHD.

12 PRINCIPLES FOR RAISING
A CHILD WITH ADHD

INTRODUCTION

Understanding ADHD

Let's face it, over the decades that the disorder has been diagnosed, ADHD has gotten a bad name. In fact, the name is part of the problem. As a label intended to convey what the problem is, "attention-deficit/hyperactivity disorder" is limited, superficial, and misleading. As a result (with some help from widespread misinformation), many among the public don't really understand what this disorder is. That's unfortunate for parents exposed to these inaccurate views, because understanding the basic nature of ADHD is a prerequisite for getting your child the appropriate treatment and, more important to the focus of this book, parenting the child successfully from day to day.

ADHD IS NOT JUST AN ATTENTION DISORDER

ADHD is not just a disorder of attention. It is essentially a disorder of self-regulation. To put it more completely, ADHD is a neurodevelopmental disorder of self-control and executive functioning. Understanding the implications of this definition unlocks the full power of the 12 principles in this book to help you raise a child or teen with ADHD successfully.

> If you've read the fourth edition of *Taking Charge of ADHD,* you're up to speed on the nature of ADHD and don't need to read this chapter except as a refresher—or to understand how each of the

dozen principles flows directly from what we know about ADHD through decades of research. I recommend that you obtain a copy of *Taking Charge of ADHD* to refer to when you want a more detailed explanation of the disorder. I also recommend Joel Nigg's *Getting Ahead of ADHD* for additional scientific background for those who are interested.

THE FUNDAMENTAL FACTS ABOUT ADHD

You'll need a solid understanding of the symptoms of ADHD and how they will likely affect your child's functioning to parent your child effectively. But first let's lay the foundation:

ADHD is a neurodevelopmental disorder. This simply means that the disorder often arises during childhood and adolescence and affects the development of the brain that occurs primarily during these years (although some brain development continues into our late 20s). Research has compared brain scans of children with ADHD and typical children over almost a decade and found that those with ADHD averaged delays in brain development of 2–3 years across that time period.

The cause is primarily genetic. Disturbances in specific genes responsible for building and operating the brain increase the risk of having ADHD in about 70% of cases. There are environmental causes as well, but they account for only a small percentage of cases. These include consumption of too much alcohol by the pregnant mother, consumption of lead (usually through lead paint) by a young child, head trauma, other brain injuries, infections, tumors, strokes, and other adverse events that clearly affect certain networks in the brain.

ADHD is defined as having more trouble than others with two groups of behaviors: (1) persisting toward goals while resisting distractions and (2) inhibiting impulsive actions. Because of common patterns in brain development, we all have some ability to pay attention, resist distractions, persist toward our goals, remember what we intend to do while going about doing it, inhibit acting on mere impulse or the first thought that enters the mind, inhibit restlessness, and restrict our activity level so it is appropriate to particular situations. These abilities can therefore be considered human traits, and each of us falls along a spectrum from typical to untypical for each trait. Those with ADHD fall on the untypical end of these spectrums—they have a lot more trouble than typical children with sustaining attention and action and are a lot more likely to be hyperactive or to have trouble controlling impulses. Our abilities in these areas also improve with age, with most children coming to do these things well enough to meet the demands and expectations of a situation appropriately for their age thanks to normal brain development. Children with ADHD, however, are significantly delayed in this pattern of development. When children develop these traits so little that they show the symptoms of ADHD and thus experience the negative consequences of functioning ineffectively in various domains of their life, the problem becomes a psychological disorder.

The box on the next page describes what this neurodevelopmental disorder looks like in one particular child; you might find the depiction somewhat familiar.

ADHD is a universal disorder affecting 5–8% of children— about 1 in every 15 to 20. ADHD affects more boys than girls at first, but then the gender divide narrows—from three times as many boys as girls in childhood to about twice as many boys in adolescence and only 1.5 as many adult males as females. The disorder is seen in all ethnic groups and social classes and has been identified in every country that has examined their children for it. This finding confirms that ADHD is primarily biological (neurodevelopmental) and not caused mainly by social or environmental factors such as culture.

The fact that this disorder is biological led naturally to many of the principles in this book, beginning with Principle 2, which encourages us to remember that ADHD is a real disorder, and continuing with the next four, all focused on helping a child who has a problem he was born with and didn't ask to have. The neurodevelopmental nature of ADHD also informs the practical principles in the second half of this book, which address the specific symptoms of ADHD.

THE SYMPTOMS OF ADHD

If your child has ADHD, you'll likely see a lot of behaviors every day that flow from two sets of highly related symptoms—problems with attention and problems with inhibition and hyperactivity. Having a lot of these

What ADHD Looks Like in One Child

Niko was just 2 years old when his mother knew that there was trouble ahead for this little whirling dervish. Never content to be still for more than a few seconds, and flitting about from one object to another in their house, it was as if he lived for one thing only—motion. Instead of walking, he would run, tumble, and jump, and just throw his body about the room. Though a happy if not silly child most of the time, as he grew older, Niko could also have meltdowns when he was frustrated or didn't get his way. Emotionally impulsive, Niko let you know where you stood with him all the time as he wore his emotions on his sleeve. And he could be exhausting, getting into everything he could find, open, unlatch, or uncover. As a result, he had three serious injuries (laceration from a can, poisoning from fluids under the sink, head injury from jumping off a boulder in the backyard) before he was 5 years old, and several more thereafter.

By the time Niko was 4, his mom, Chris, discovered he couldn't snuggle for very long while watching TV. And mealtimes were a circus, as Niko would take a bite of food, run about the kitchen, climb back in his chair for another quick bite, then rock his chair back, often tipping it over and then crawling under the table to pet the family dog. His preschool teacher complained that she nearly always had to have one hand on him to contain him while supervising and teaching the other children. And sitting still for longer than a minute or two during story or "carpet" (teaching) time was next to impossible. Complicating matters further, his teacher reported that he "never shuts up." He had a comment about everything but listened to no one, a problem Chris had seen many times at home. His teacher even advised Chris that Niko should stay back a year and not start kindergarten with the other children as he simply didn't have the academic readiness behaviors that make children available for learning: sustaining attention, inhibiting irrelevant activity, and remembering and complying with instructions. That's when Chris took Niko to the pediatrician to insist that he refer them to a specialist in children's behavior and development. After a child psychologist spent several hours evaluating Niko, Chris had her answer as to what was going wrong—ADHD.

problems and showing them often is important to the diagnosis: a child who shows only some of these problems, and only occasionally, would fall closer to the "typical" end of the spectrum and not be diagnosed with ADHD. To qualify for the diagnosis, your child has to have shown these problems for 6 months, in two or more domains of life, to a much greater degree than other children, and they have to be causing problems with functioning in major life activities, such as in school, home life, or peer relationships.

Problems with Attention

Children with ADHD often:

- Appear not to listen to what is being said
- Fail to finish assigned tasks
- Lose things, especially those things needed to complete tasks
- Can't concentrate as well as other children
- Are easily distracted
- Have problems working without supervision
- Require more redirection
- Shift from one uncompleted activity to another
- Can't recall what they were told to do or should be doing in a given situation

Problems with Inhibition

Of course, children with ADHD are also likely to have problems with being impulsive. They often:

- Interrupt or intrude on others and what the others are doing
- Talk excessively, often speaking or acting out of turn
- Don't think about what they are doing before they do it, acting too quickly on impulse
- Have difficulty waiting for things and postponing self-gratification

▤ Opt to do things that provide immediate gratification or rewards, even when inappropriate

▤ Display their emotions very quickly, too strongly, and with little effort to moderate them so that they are more appropriate for a situation—especially negative emotions such as impatience, frustration, hostility, temper, anger, or even aggression when provoked

> It can be heartbreaking to watch your child struggle with emotional control. Even when the emotions they feel are perfectly normal in a given situation, children with ADHD often react more quickly and extremely than other kids their age. As a result they often end up rejected or avoided by their peers.

▤ Fail to anticipate the consequences of risky behavior and proceed full speed ahead, ending up with far more accidental injuries of all sorts than other children, more sports injuries—and end up visiting the ER at least three times more often than others and usually with more severe injuries

Problems with Excessive or "Hyper" Activity

Related to this problem with inhibition is one of excessive activity level, or hyperactivity. Children with ADHD often:

▤ Act as if driven by a motor, moving about a room or setting much more than others, being nearly constantly in motion

▤ Are restless, fidgety, and "squirmy," moving their arms and legs about while trying mightily to keep their butts in the chair when required to sit still

▤ Touch things or even others

▤ Act more forcefully and abruptly than others and engage more than others in excessive movements

▤ Talk more than others, making more vocal sounds or noises in general than others their age

▤ Climb on things excessively when young, running about a room or play area more than others and engaging in all sorts of attention-seeking antics

■ Get into things, especially inappropriate things, more than other children and so have to be supervised much more often and more closely than other children

How Severe the Symptoms Are May Depend on the Situation

I said above that your child's symptoms have to appear frequently and in at least two different domains of life (such as at home and at school) to be diagnosed as ADHD, but that doesn't mean they'll be as severe in every setting. Symptoms of ADHD may often be worse in settings or tasks that:

■ Are boring or uninteresting

■ Involve significantly delayed consequences or infrequent feedback

■ Require working independently of others

■ Lack supervision

■ Involve groups of children

■ Are highly familiar (and thus usually less interesting)

■ Involve parents rather than strangers or less familiar adults

■ Include parents or supervisors who talk and reason too much and rarely act to control misbehavior

■ Require waiting

■ Occur late in the afternoon or evening (due to fatigue in self-control)

■ Place substantial restrictions on movement (like classroom desk work!)

Maybe you've already noticed that these are the situations that typically demand self-regulation. And perhaps you've already seen that your child's symptoms are often milder in situations that don't require a lot of self-regulation. These could be situations that involve fun activities, highly stimulating or interesting tasks (e.g., video games, cartoons, animated movies), lots of movement (e.g., gym, recess, sports), frequent rewards or feedback, lots of supervision, working in small teams with peers rather than independently, working one-on-one with an adult, highly novel settings, supervisors who speak briefly but back up their rules with consequences, and little or no pressure to wait for things. That's because these types of situations don't demand much from your child's executive functions.

THE EXECUTIVE IN YOUR CHILD'S BRAIN

The symptoms of ADHD described above are really just its surface features—the outward manifestations of an underlying complex problem in psychological development. Those symptoms arise from a set of underlying mental abilities or brain functions called the *executive functions*. They are called "executive" because they act in ways that organize the rest of the brain to accomplish our goals and plans. Executive functions really are all about being able to regulate our own behavior with an eye to the future and accomplishing our goals. Not surprisingly, the same networks in the brain are involved in both ADHD and executive functioning: the networks that permit us to decide to focus, make a game plan, stay on task, move and think efficiently, and choose what's important to pay attention to and act on from among all the competing inputs in any environment.

Most neuropsychologists believe that these networks (and others) give rise to at least seven executive functions that interact to allow us to control our own behavior using hindsight and foresight to anticipate and prepare for the future. They mostly occur in the frontal part of the brain, behind your forehead. But the networks in which they are involved extend to many other parts of the brain. The impact of the executive function deficits involved in ADHD are just as far-reaching. You'll see them in many aspects of your child's behavior, in many domains of daily life. Like an executive in a business, the executive in the brain contemplates the future, develops plans, and determines how best to operate at the moment to ensure current *and later* survival, success, and well-being. So a child with ADHD might behave in ways that are detrimental to him right now (by impulsively leaping out of his chair at school) and in the future (by not understanding that doing well in school could cause him problems far into the future). As you'll see in the following descriptions, these executive functions don't operate individually but together, further increasing the effect they have on how any individual thinks, feels, and acts.

This frontal part of the brain is where goals get invented and plans to achieve those goals are formulated. It also sees to it that the plan is put into action, is monitored for progress, and is adjusted as needed to accomplish the goal. Executive functions help a child grow up to become an independent, self-determining person who can make and pursue plans successfully. Without them, we would all bounce from impulse to impulse with little direction toward any goal we might want to reach.

Executive Function 1: Self-Awareness

Self-control begins with knowing what you're thinking, saying, and doing. Fortunately for all of us, a lot of what we do is automatic, part of well-learned patterns of behavior. But sometimes priorities change or the unexpected occurs and we have to override autopilot. This fundamental executive function allows us to monitor our actions to see how well we are doing at getting to our goals (or those assigned to us by others).

Children and teens with ADHD are less able to watch over what they are thinking, saying, feeling, and doing and end up running on automatic pilot even when circumstances arise that require a course correction—they can't see as well as their peers that autopilot isn't getting them where they need to go. This makes the child with ADHD more distractible and reactive to events playing out inside and around her rather than being more proactive, thoughtful, and deliberate. Like a driverless car, she careens around life bouncing off guardrails, speeding recklessly, and running through the warning lights and stop signs of life because she isn't paying much attention to what she's doing.

In our social world, self-control and thoughtful, deliberate action are prized because they promote actions that are best for our own long-term welfare and less likely to conflict with those of others. Without self-awareness, a child will have trouble being thoughtful or deliberate. That's why following Principle 6 can be helpful. When you understand why your child isn't as able to monitor what he's doing as well as other kids his age, you can get in the habit of supporting development of this lagging executive function.

Executive Function 2: Inhibition or Self-Restraint

Thoughtful, goal-directed actions also require the child to inhibit the impulse to keep acting without thinking first. Inhibition and self-restraint create that all-important pause between what happens in the environment and your child's response to it. That pause gives the child time to think, and that thinking makes him proactive rather than always reactive to events. In that tiny space your child can choose among various courses of action to improve the likelihood of something better happening later (getting a larger payoff or avoiding a greater harm)—in 5 minutes, tomorrow, the next week, the next month, and even years ahead.

A child who has trouble controlling impulses may seem to those who have this ability to be thoughtless, heedless, ill advised, and even irrational or at least immature. But when you know that the problem is rooted in a lagging ability to inhibit impulses, you can help your child focus when necessary and also stop focusing on one thing when necessary. Principles 6–8 can guide you in helping your child create the necessary pause that leads to better choices. And because underdeveloped inhibition can be a particular problem when you're away from home, Principle 12 is the rule to follow to anticipate problems and head them off.

As you may know, children with ADHD don't just jump from task to task; sometimes they "hyperfocus" on something that's fun or immediately gratifying, to the detriment of tasks they have to shift to (at school, for example). So the child with ADHD keeps playing the video game he started when he woke up this morning instead of getting ready for school or shifting to a task at home he agreed to do, such as Saturday morning chores. Or a child refuses to leave the water park where a birthday party is being held, or keeps binge-watching an exciting TV series instead of starting homework. Or she stays on social media when she should be getting ready for soccer practice and ends up late. The principles noted above can help in all of these circumstances. Principle 6 will help you teach your child to be accountable regarding when to inhibit behavior.

Executive Function 3: Working Memory

We all have a GPS-like device (a network) in our brain that allows us to call up maps of our past (hindsight) and use them to contemplate a goal or destination and then pursue that goal (foresight). It's called your working memory, and like your GPS, it really has two parts, one that uses images (maps) and another that tells you verbally how to get where you are going in the most efficient way. These two components of working memory interact to help us remember what we're supposed to be doing and guide us toward our goals. Working memory holds information (images and instructions) that we will use to guide us to our desired destination, monitor our progress, and even suggest alternative routes (problem solving) if we encounter obstacles along the way.

Working memory is different from long-term storage of information. Basically, it is remembering so as to do something, and those with ADHD are not necessarily forgetting information but rather forgetting what they're supposed to be doing in this place at this time. Imagine your daughter going into a bedroom to get dressed for school. She sees her tablet on her bed, recalls that she was going to text a friend about where to meet her outside the school, and does that instead. She forgets to dress, and so 20 minutes later when it's time to leave the house for the bus she is still in her pajamas. Any distraction or stimulus around her, like her smartphone or tablet, is far more powerful at capturing her attention than her memory of the task she is supposed to be doing. Children with ADHD seem to be governed by the environment around them rather than the ideas they had or the instructions they were given about what they were going to do.

One way that this forgetfulness can show up is when children with ADHD don't follow through on directives, rules, promises, instructions, or commitments the way others are able to do. Of course, part of this is due to their inattention—they weren't listening when they were told what to do—but in many cases it's problematic working memory: they cannot hold in mind just what rules, instructions, or promises they are supposed to be acting on. Mental representations, like rules or instructions, are simply not powerful enough to guide behavior in those with ADHD as they do in others. That's why one thing parents and others can do to help is to make these rules and other directives concrete and visible—see Principle 9. Your child will also need more reminders of what to do (and not do) than other kids, and these should involve more gentle touch and tangible rewards than verbal commands—see Principle 7.

Learning in childhood and adolescence and also functioning in the adult world depend on the ability to hold multiple pieces of related information in the mind, to connect the dots using our working memory. So naturally deficits in this executive function can take a toll on academic achievement and ultimately success in the workplace. Principle 9 is all about boosting working memory, and you'll find detailed, up-to-date information on academic supports in the fourth edition of *Taking Charge of ADHD*.

Executive Function 4:
A Sense of Time and Time Management

Children and teens with ADHD are essentially blind to time. They can't seem to sense and use the passage of time in controlling their own behavior as well as others. So they don't get things done on time, in time, over time. They fail to prepare for deadlines, to understand how long it may take to do things or how much time they need to get somewhere they need to go. They also seem clueless about the future more generally. Thus, they do not think about the future consequences of their actions *before* they happen. Thinking about future consequences requires both working memory and a sense of time passing and of the probable future itself. Those last two things represent hindsight and foresight—things that children and teens with ADHD don't seem to use much when deciding on how to act.

All that seems to matter to those with ADHD is "the now." So they are typically late for work, appointments, deadlines, classes, and meetings. They often do not keep time commitments they make with others, and school assignments are turned in late or not at all. The child, and especially the teen, with ADHD is not prepared when deadlines finally do arrive. Your child may wait until the last minute when the future has now arrived and then try scrambling to do what should have been done much earlier. He may simply not do the work at all once he realizes it's too late to complete it.

In the diagram on the facing page you can see how a child's sense of the future typically expands as the child matures. But the child with ADHD still has a relatively narrow window onto time and can't think as far ahead. Fortunately, you (and others) can help your child see a more distant horizon. See Principle 8.

Executive Function 5: Emotional Self-Control

Life is filled with frustrating and anger-inducing events, especially for a child. Those events can strongly provoke our emotions. When such emotionally charged events occur, children with ADHD are likely to react quickly with their primary initial emotions rather than showing some emotional restraint. They fail to think through the situation more carefully, don't moderate their strong emotions, and don't try to substitute a more socially acceptable emotional reaction that is good for them in the

The Development of Foresight: An Emerging Window on Time

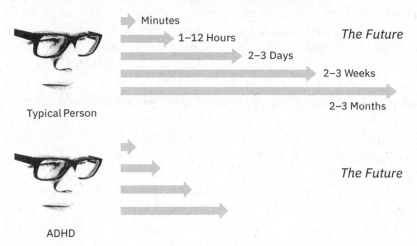

long run. Instead, children and teens with ADHD seem to "wear their emotions on their sleeve" for all to see when they are provoked by events or by others around them.

As noted above, the consequences can be heartbreaking to witness. You know that your child isn't being self-centered, demanding, or intentionally aggressive. Others may not; they just avoid your child. They don't know that children with ADHD lack the working memory to use images of positive past experiences and the impulse control to talk themselves into calming down before reacting inappropriately. But now you know, and you can use the guidance in this book to remind yourself when things get heated that your child has a disorder—it's not a matter of "won't" but of "can't." See Principles 2–4, which I've found crucial in establishing and maintaining the compassionate, supportive, but authoritative (not authoritarian!) mindset needed to raise a child with ADHD and keep your home a sanctuary for the whole family.

Executive Function 6: Self-Motivation

When faced with routine chores or tasks or other boring activities, children with ADHD often lack the self-motivation to get things done, instead seeking more interesting, exciting, or rewarding things to do. Many children with ADHD are sensation seekers, looking for anything to do that gives them some short-term burst of arousal or entertainment. Teens with ADHD speed far more than other adolescent drivers and participate more often in dangerous activities like extreme sports (speed skiing, skydiving, extreme snowboarding, car racing, motorcycle use or racing, etc.). They also sometimes over- or hyperfocus on and may even become addicted to playing sensational Internet video games. But even things that are initially interesting to them may lose their appeal over time, and this happens much faster than it does in others. Their lives are filled with half-completed projects that seemed like good ideas at the time but lost their appeal very quickly.

Being blind to time can also interfere with motivation, at least with longer-term goals. Children with ADHD will not appreciate the larger, later, and more important consequences in life as much as the smaller, more obvious ones in the moment. And so they won't bother to work as long and as hard to get the rewards that are further out in the future. Without extra incentives to do so, they will usually choose the immediate gratifications offered over the ones they have to wait for. Without additional supports, children with ADHD will have trouble with sharing, cooperation, turn taking, and also with repaying the favors of others or fulfilling promises made to others. Principles 6 and 7 will help you apply such supports and even devise new ones that suit your family's unique needs.

Being able to share, cooperate, and reciprocate depends on our capacities for self-restraint, self-awareness, foresight, and deferred gratification. Without those executive functions, kids with ADHD aren't motivated to do things for others just because family, friends, and later coworkers and colleagues will be more likely to do the same for them down the road. The deficiencies in the executive system of the brain in ADHD can help us understand why maturing children with ADHD may be having more problems in their family, social world, school, and, later as teens, in their driving, work, and even financial life than others. Principle 2 will help you remind yourself that ADHD is a disorder.

Executive Function 7:
Self-Organization, Planning, and Problem Solving

Because children, and particularly teens, with ADHD are so easily distracted by events around them, more easily bored, and less able to keep paying attention to what they planned to do or should be doing, they leave a trail of disorganization in their wake. They drop things where they were last used rather than consciously putting them back where they belong, such as placing schoolbooks and homework in their backpack, placing the bag by the door, or, for teens, placing car keys on a hook by the back door. They often leave dirty dishes and food wrappers throughout the house, misplace money or other valuables like smartphones, or forget to charge them—even if they can find their charger. Those with ADHD cannot sustain their actions toward goals so that the goals are completed, and they wind up filling lockers and desks and closets with lots of unfinished projects. All of this makes for a messy, cluttered, and disorganized life at home and in school—but Principle 10 can help.

Related to this problem with self-organization is a difficulty with planning and problem solving. Planning and problem solving involve the ability to generate multiple ideas or options for how to respond to a current problem (an obstacle to our goals) or to an impending future event. It is a form of creativity. It also involves thinking about how best to sequence the steps we may eventually choose to use to accomplish that goal. It is a type of mental play that comes from the ability to take apart and recombine information in our mind. And it is much harder to do if your mind and life are poorly organized, as they are in the developing child and teen with ADHD.

People with ADHD simply don't plan things out or problem-solve very well. Consequently, we hear them complain that not just their life but their mind is a jumbled, poorly organized mess, and they are less able to use it effectively to hold information in working memory. And we hear teens with ADHD complain that they cannot manipulate that information quickly to plan out possible courses of action or to problem-solve their way around obstacles as well as others. This deficiency will have a substantial adverse effect on their social and educational activities in particular, where mental problem solving is so essential to success. Again, Principle 9 can help with working memory, and Principles 10 and 11 can help you support your child's efforts to plan and problem-solve effectively.

WHAT TO DO ABOUT IT?

Recognizing these deficits in executive functioning should help you understand why ADHD is such a serious disorder. The executive deficits underlying ADHD impair the ability to become independent of our parents and

Is ADHD a Gift?[1]

Is there a positive side to having ADHD? Some writers have represented ADHD as a gift and continue to do so. They see it as bringing advantages (such as creativity) that those without the disorder would not possess. Now that you've read about the neurodevelopmental roots of ADHD, the symptoms, and the executive function problems ADHD causes, you might find it somewhat absurd to portray this disorder as a gift. I believe portraying ADHD as an advantage of some sort is a mistake. First of all, it misrepresents the scientific findings—none of the thousands of science articles published on ADHD have found the disorder to confer some special advantage, talent, ability, or other trait on those who have it. Second, it minimizes the seriousness of the disorder and can also foster false hope. Worst of all, it can deny children needed help since "gifts" don't require treatment.

If ADHD were such a great thing to have, why should society provide special accommodations and services in school or college for those who have it? Why should such a "gift" make an adult with ADHD eligible for worker's compensation or Social Security disability payments? Why should children who have it be granted special protections against discrimination in school under Section 504 of the Americans with Disabilities Act? Why should insurance companies help pay for visits to mental health professionals and treatments for it? You can see the problem here. ADHD cannot be both a gift and a serious disability. It cannot be something commendable while also be deserving of society's compassion and help. Your child deserves that compassion and help, and so do you.

---

[1]*Note.* Adapted and modified from similar material in my book *When an Adult You Love Has ADHD* (APA LifeTools, Washington, DC, 2016).

others—to develop self-control, self-care, and self-determination. Those abilities are critical for planning, organizing, and carrying out behavior over time to accomplish goals (and other work) so as to be well prepared for the future.

The remainder of this book sets forth the principles that can help you address or at least accommodate these executive deficits. In each chapter I explain the essential problem to be addressed and then offer solutions specifically targeted to that problem. These principles don't just tell you what to do or how to do it; like this introduction, they are intended to provide the "why" of what needs to be done to help your child be as independent and successful as possible. Over many years of working with parents and their children with ADHD, I've found that having a deeper understanding of what the problem is and why a problem exists can stimulate much greater insight into what to do than just being handed a list of instructions. Once you know the reasons—the principles behind the solutions—you can invent new methods to address the problems you face. After all, your child is unique, and so is your life. In my experience, having principles to guide you to what to do in the many situations that will arise will make you a better, more effective parent than just having a book of recipes to follow without knowing why you need to use them. It's my hope and belief that this book will help you raise a child who is healthy, happy, and successful—even with the challenge of ADHD.

PRINCIPLE

1

USE THE KEYS TO SUCCESS

All parents want their children to grow into successful adults. Each of us may define success slightly differently, but it's likely that we all hope our children will grow up to be independent, responsible, self-supporting, and content. The question, when ADHD is in the mix, is how to get them there. As you've just read in the Introduction, ADHD comes with a group of challenges that at times may make your child's prospects of achieving success seem somewhat dim. The impulsiveness, inattention, disorganization, deficient emotional control, and other effects of executive function deficits can make it difficult for your child to make good choices in the moment and plan for a good future, whether that's later today or 10 years from now. How can your son or daughter get around these challenges?

> **THE PROBLEM:** It's very hard to predict outcomes for children with ADHD with any precision—but the absence of a few key factors will make growing into a successful adult much more difficult.

Follow-up studies of children with ADHD into adulthood suggest to some extent that better outcomes are linked to:

- Greater intelligence
- More education
- Milder symptoms of ADHD
- The absence of any other psychological disorders

- ■ Better family socioeconomic circumstances
- ■ Having a two-parent household
- ■ Better neighborhoods
- ■ More friends in childhood

If you looked at that list and thought these factors are probably help-ful to all children while they're growing up, you'd be right. And although they were found to be weak predictors of positive outcomes for those with ADHD and certainly weren't the keys to success for everyone, they might have some benefits for your child. But in my decades of experience with families I've found that having parents who are active advocates for their children, who recognize that their children have a disorder and need extra support, and who eagerly focus on their children's strengths is a more important and fundamentally huge benefit.

ADHD is not a gift. It does not usually confer any benefits, blessings, unusual talents, or superior traits. It can lead to a shorter life expectancy by as much as 12 years if not treated in adulthood due to the propensities it causes for poor health maintenance, diet, sleep, exercise, and an excessive use of tobacco and alcohol. It can be a serious and even life-threatening disorder that if unmanaged can double the risk of early death in childhood and more than quadruple it in adulthood. Yet its symptoms may interact with other talents or gifts of the individual, as well as high intelligence, a supportive family or social environment, treatment, and special resources so as to promote success.

And there definitely are success stories among adults with ADHD. Many of them, unfortunately, tend to focus on just one aspect of their life, such as the vocation in which they are unusually successful. Those stories often ignore the other domains of life in which they may be struggling, such as socially, financially, legally, in their intimate relationships, and in their substance use. On the other hand, a closer look at these success-ful adults often reveals that they're doing well today because they have had supportive loved ones surrounding them, particularly their parents. In fact, I have come to believe that the role of their loved ones is absolutely critical to the success of children with ADHD.

A notable example of how important this kind of support and dedica-tion is comes from Olympic swimmer Michael Phelps, whose mother and sisters helped him:

- Channel his energies
- Focus and develop his athletic talent
- Find area resources that could further develop his athletic gifts
- Buffer him from the difficulties he was having with school and provide him with more individualized academic assistance
- Support him financially and emotionally
- Keep him so involved and organized that there simply was little if any time for him to get into trouble most days

It undoubtedly helped Michael at school that his mother was an assistant principal and had taught school herself for several decades. And so when he was not doing so well she worked with Michael herself as well as getting him extra attention in school to address his severe problems with concentration. She also hired a tutor for him in math when he struggled with it, used sports examples to help him learn to solve word problems in math, and got him a separate seat arrangement in school when he kept bothering other children. She also developed cuing strategies to help him control his emotions, especially his temper, when he did not do well in swim meets. In general, she advises parents to work as a team with their children and teens with ADHD to help them through their difficulties with handling work and life challenges.

Michael has been very clear about how important his family, especially his mother, was to his success. He repeatedly and publicly acknowledges his gratitude to his mother, sisters, and coach for their involvement in his success. If Michael is any example, the loved ones around people with ADHD clearly can have a constructive influence on them.

And Michael Phelps is just one example, as evidenced by the thousands of other children and adults with ADHD who may not have achieved this level of success (yet!) but who are definitely thriving.

Consider Phillip, whose parents sought my help when he was about to be kicked out of third grade at a neighborhood parochial school because of his chronic inability to concentrate on his work, refrain from being the class clown, and sit still during lectures by the teachers and nuns running the school. It was their devotion to their son and their diligence in figuring out what would help him succeed that set Phillip on the path toward better functioning. After experimenting with various medications, we determined that a nonstimulant (Strattera) was best for him given the side effects he experienced on the more traditional ADHD stimulant medications. To that we added a daily behavior report card (which you will learn about later in this book) that was linked to a home reward program, along with afterschool one-on-one tutoring twice weekly with a retired special education teacher who worked part-time as a private tutor. These interventions were just enough to allow this otherwise intelligent child to graduate from this elementary school, later attend the local college prep parochial high school, and go on to Auburn University, where he majored in biology. He now travels throughout the mid-Atlantic region as a water specialist with the regional environmental protection agency, testing the various lakes, streams, reservoirs, and other water resources for their environmental quality.

Pearl, too, was lucky enough to have parents who pursued all the options available to help her overcome her poor grades in school and incessant penchant for socializing with other teens at times when she should have been doing schoolwork, studying, or paying attention to teacher lectures. Pearl's parents brought her to our ADHD clinic, and she responded well to the ADHD stimulant medication we prescribed, along with special educational assistance and accommodations in school for her handwriting and organizational deficits. Even then she was only an average student, yet she graduated high school, took a community college series of courses in event planning, and now works in the sales branch of a large event planning company that organizes business conferences. Her talent for interacting with others, enthusiasm for her work, desire to travel as part of her life, and gift for starting conversations with anyone she meets all combined to make her ideal as a salesperson for this company. It was her parents who helped us see the strengths that Pearl had. Yet she also attributed some of her career success to having gotten the company to hire an administrative assistant who is highly organized but socially reclusive and is happy to work in a corporate office cubicle handling the paperwork and scheduling needed to follow up on the sales contracts that Pearl obtained.

And then there is Daleena, who, like most children with ADHD, was doing poorly in her schoolwork and also quite disruptive of the family's home life when she did not get her way, which was often. Her parents attended our parent behavior management training course and were able to quell this drift of their daughter toward oppositional behavior. Rather than employ medication, they opted to have the daughter enrolled in a small private school nearby that specialized in children with learning and attentional disorders and provided much smaller student-to-teacher ratios. As she grew up, Daleena showed a fascination for crime dramas on cable television and loved the problem-solving nature of the work she observed. Her parents encouraged her to enroll in a community college medical program for lab techs during which she also interned at a local hospital pathology lab. There she met people who helped her parlay her talents into working for the city police laboratory doing the lab tests and some of the actual field work required to gather the evidence that buttressed police investigations.

Would these individuals with ADHD have gotten where they are today without the diligent attention and support of their parents? I doubt it. I've seen so many examples of children blossoming when their parents sought the best treatment and accommodations for their children and also helped the professionals working with their children recognize and capitalize on the children's strengths. Most of the children and teens with ADHD that I've worked with needed just the right tailoring of a treatment package of medication, educational support, alternative educational routes, parent training in child behavior management, family support, and cultivation of talents to become independent, self-supporting adults. What their stories illustrate is that parents need to persevere and often think outside the box.

THE SOLUTION: Four keys to success.

Looking closely at the role of loved ones—especially parents—in the lives of children with ADHD led directly to the 12 principles in this book. But it also helped me identify four keys to success that serve as their foundation:

🔑 Get a professional evaluation, diagnosis, and treatment.

+

🔑 Identify and promote special talents and aptitudes.

+

🔑 Find community resources to develop them further.

+

🔑 Believe in, accept, and support your child with ADHD.

Key 1: Be Sure Your Child Has Been Professionally Evaluated, Diagnosed, and Treated

ADHD can be treated effectively. And your child is far more likely to succeed in life with the help of such treatment. The first step toward ensuring success for your child is to get a thorough professional evaluation so that appropriate treatments can be initiated, whether that's FDA-approved medications or any of the other evidence-based treatments for managing ADHD, from classroom behavior management methods to special educational services and behavioral parent training programs. Optimal results are typically obtained from a combination of treatments instead of just individual ones. Implementing the principles in this book will also take you a long way toward success for your child. (See the fourth edition of *Taking Charge of ADHD* for details on diagnosis and treatment, plus behavior management in school and at home as well as accommodations at school. The fundamentals of behavior management methods also appear throughout this book.)

The benefits of appropriate treatment were once summed up by TV star and artist Ty Pennington, whose penchant for destroying things and rebuilding them as a child evolved into a popular television show, *Extreme Makeover: Home Edition*. "Now . . . I can actually complete the tasks. I can actually finish a sentence and actually finish the projects that I've got on my to-do list. Once I was put on long-lasting medications like Vyvanse, next thing you know, bam, it's like somebody gave me glasses and all of a sudden I could see, not only what I couldn't see before but I could see the mistakes I made and how I could correct them." About his success in art school he added, "My grades went from Ds to As; instead of doing one project, I'm actually *completing* three, could show just how talented I am."

Ty Pennington is one among many with ADHD who have found a career that takes advantage of their strengths and preferences. But in virtually all cases they would never have gotten there without proper treatment as children and teenagers. As a teen, Marilana loved the family's trips to garage and yard sales, out-of-the-way antiques businesses, and estate auctions. She developed a fascination for toys, books, and household appliances from earlier decades and proved to have quite an eye for items with value that could be resold for a profit. Despite this talent, Marilana always struggled in school even with high intelligence. Indeed, her IQ was part of her problem, as her school balked at providing her with appropriate special education accommodations and assistance, believing her to be just a bored, troublesome, yet gifted student and not someone with ADHD. After much discussion, her parents and I agreed to have Marilana tried on an ADHD medication but, more importantly, to transfer her to a private school specializing in learning disabilities and ADHD. Marilana had four successful years at this special school and went on to a nearby small university to obtain a liberal arts degree. She now works as a partner in a rare books dealership that allows her to travel the world searching for rare books and meeting with potential clients for the books her agency has obtained. This story is another example of how parental persistence got a child the help she really needed, despite doubts by the school system.

Most schools do the best they can for their students. But ADHD poses challenges for some, especially when resources are limited. Levon's parents didn't know where to turn when the administrators and teachers at his rural school decided that his problems with attention and completion of schoolwork were attributable to lax discipline from his parents rather than a neurodevelopmental condition. When they brought Levon to see me for an evaluation, and I diagnosed him with ADHD, we decided together to try medication. This treatment was reasonably successful, but Levon could have benefited from accommodations and support at school as well. It quickly became evident that they would not be provided, because the school preferred to expend its meager special education resources on clearly intellectually and physically disabled students rather than on children with learning or behavioral problems. It was clear that getting Levon through this school system would be difficult, but I encouraged the parents to accept the fact that our limited goal was getting the child through school by any means even if it meant with mediocre grades. With the dedicated support of his parents and the boost he got from medication, Levon did make it through, and today he is successfully employed in work he loves. As a child Levon loved to explore the outdoors, and he had plenty of opportunities to ramble around the area's forests, rivers, ponds, and lakes. Happiest when roaming freely outdoors, he took a surveying course at a technical college and not only did well with the math but enjoyed the exploration and mapping of the regional terrain that this profession provided. Although he graduated from high school with barely a C average, he is now a partner in a small surveying company and an independent adult. Again, no small thanks are due his parents, who waged a constant battle against the conservative, old-fashioned views about disorders like ADHD that they were surrounded by.

Key 2: Identify Your Child's Talents and Aptitudes

As the preceding stories attest, one key to success for many individuals with ADHD is identifying an aptitude or talent in which that child also has a strong interest. Because executive skill deficits often stand in the way of more obvious career paths, this is commonly a nontraditional or unconventional pursuit. Parents therefore need to be astute in their knowledge of their unique child.

Athletics are a particularly good example—although far from the only one—as we can see in the example of Michael Phelps. Phelps seems to have inherited some of his athletic talent, but people with ADHD also may be more likely to function effectively (to be less impaired) in physical education or sports than might be the case in other educational majors. This is known in psychology as "niche picking," and we all do it. Over time, we learn where we are likely to succeed and fail given our strengths, weaknesses, and interests. So we keep self-selecting into those pursuits where we seem to do OK or in which we excel, while avoiding other pursuits in which we have no talent, no history of success, and probably some experience with failure.

Activities that involve exercise are also doubly beneficial for children with ADHD because routine exercise helps them manage and reduce their symptoms after exercise and may combat their higher risk for obesity. This may be why we have such a long list of successful athletes with ADHD; see the box on the facing page.

Niche Picking

You may already have some idea of where your child with ADHD shines. But here's a list of questions to consider so as to identify niches for success:

- What are your child's strengths?
- What are your child's inherent interests?
- Apart from any academic talents, is your child good at . . .
  - Music
  - Visual arts
  - Performing arts
  - Photography or videography

Successful Athletes with ADHD (among Many Others)

Golfers Bubba Watson and the late Payne Stewart

Gymnasts Louis Smith and Simone Biles

Judo competitor Ashley McKenzie

Football star and commentator Terry Bradshaw

Football players Andre Brown and Virgil Green

Baseball stars Shane Victorino, Andrés Torres, and Pete Rose

Track star Justin Gatlin

Hockey player Cammi Granato

Competitive rower Adam Kreek

Professional basketball players Michael Jordan and Chris Kaman

Olympic decathlete Bruce (now Caitlyn) Jenner

Cyclist and Tour de France winner Greg LeMond

Professional wrestler Matt Morgan

- Technology
- Mechanics
- Culinary arts
- Outdoor recreational activities
- Sports
- Any of the trades
- Sales or persuasiveness
- Entrepreneurship or self-employment

Parents have often been surprised to discover an unknown talent in their children that they could channel into a true strength. So be openminded about unusual aptitudes in your child that you might not think could be used for a successful vocation. But keep in mind that this doesn't have to mean something that will turn your child into an elite athlete, a virtuoso performer, or a business tycoon. It can be any small interest or strength into which your child can channel energy. Find out what your child's interest or talent is and then use the next key to success to help it blossom.

As examples, over my years in clinical practice I have had cases involving:

- A boy who fixed electric motors for other kids' radio-controlled cars who went on to technical school to learn to be an electrician and then opened his own small machine repair businesses

- A girl who loved taking pictures, first with a digital camera and then with her smartphone, whose eye for detail, angles, and meaning in her pictures garnered her awards in local and regional photography contests, despite the fact that she could barely attain passing grades in school. She eventually graduated, though a year behind her peers, and now has her own photography business specializing in shooting pictures and video at destination weddings in the United States and Europe

- A boy who rewired his bedroom light switch to turn on not just his light but also his music player, a string of chili pepper lights hung around his room, and his television, and who went on to attend engineering school and get a good job with the regional power company

- A teen who routinely explored the outdoors surrounding his home, looking for various insects and their nests, who went on to get a degree in environmental sciences and now works as a partner in a local exterminating company

- A girl whose doodling pictures were so incredibly realistic she was encouraged by her teacher to study art and now has her own studio in the arts district of a southern city

- A boy with both ADHD and dyslexia who dropped out of high school, became an assistant on board a swordfishing boat, and in his spare time drew watercolor sketches of fish, boats, and men working the boats—pictures that caught the eye of a fishing magazine editor who used them on magazine covers, thus launching his career as a very successful nature artist in an oceanside town

■ A girl whose voice even as a child was so beautifully mature her parents invested in voice lessons for her with a local voice coach that led her to sing in local restaurants as a child and go on to major in voice at a small arts college, who now works as a backup singer in a Los Angeles recording studio

■ A girl who was obsessed with and exceptional at a variety of sports as a child but had little interest in school, who went on to major in physical education at a small midwestern university and now teaches PE in a high school

■ A girl who favored cooking over homework as a teen, went on to train in culinary arts, and now has a successful website and blog about cooking, where she posts her own highly original recipes that she has compiled into successful niche cookbooks

■ A boy who was incredibly big for his age and as a teen just happened to be invited to try his hand at rugby, fell in love with the sport, and now coaches a men's rugby team that is touring in the United Kingdom

■ A boy who built structures in his backyard out of scrap wood and metal he found around his neighborhood and then pursued training in carpentry and welding at a technical college, who now owns a small business that builds tiny houses and converts shipping containers for people who want second homes on land they own in a western mountain range

■ A girl whose love of recorded music turned into a fascination with how instruments and vocals were combined to create her favorite songs, who as a teenager became an apprentice to a sound production rental company that subsequently hired her to set up equipment for various famous musicians performing in her Texas university town

There are endless such accounts of children with ADHD with nontraditional aptitudes and interests whose parents helped them enhance and expand those talents into rewarding careers. Does your child have an aptitude or interest that you could help cultivate? Perhaps your child would be inspired by the success of the individuals listed in the box on the next page.

Other Celebrities with ADHD

Every child who overcomes ADHD to succeed is a star, but your child (and you) might be inspired to know how many celebrities have ADHD: chef Jamie Oliver; dancer Karina Smirnoff (*Dancing with the Stars*); actor Will Smith; comedian/actor/artist Jim Carrey; socialite/heiress/reality TV star Paris Hilton; actor Christopher Knight (*The Brady Bunch*); TV and radio host and commentator Glenn Beck; comedian/TV host Howie Mandel; political consultant and commentator James Carville; TV star Michelle Rodriguez (*Lost*); actor/director/writer Ryan Gosling; actor Woody Harrelson; actress Mariette Hartley; singer/performer Britney Spears; singer/producer will.i.am; and singer Solange Knowles (also little sister to Beyoncé).

Key 3: Find Area Resources
That Can Help Develop That Talent

Whether your child has a real gift for a particular area of interest or a simple passion for some activity, success often depends on more than parents' support. Just being good at or interested in something isn't enough if it isn't promoted through practice, expert instruction, and more practice. Fortunately, there are many ways to identify and then open the various doors that exist to further opportunities for your child to succeed and to further enhance the child's inherent talents and aptitudes. Start looking around your community or even farther afield to find resources that can help develop your child's native talents:

- Clubs: Scouts and hobby-focused clubs can be found in most communities.

- Mentors: Ask the guidance counselor at your child's school or approach someone who has proficiency in your child's area of interest.

- Coaches: Schools, gyms, Little League, and the like are possible sources of coaches who could work with your child if sports are an interest.

- Tutors: Schools offer tutoring and also referrals to private tutors, and most communities have paid and volunteer organizations that offer tutoring.

- Retail shops that offer classes: Everything from knitting to snorkeling may be available.

- Athletic facilities: Think YMCA, Boys and Girls Clubs, and public park facilities.

- Arts councils: Most communities have one.

- Vocational technical high schools and colleges.

- Apprenticeships in local businesses.

And don't hesitate to engage any extra help that may be available to promote success in school as well. While I downplay that area of talent, as it is not a strong suit for many children with ADHD, it can be for some. (Remember Levon, described above? Once he was at technical school learning surveying, it turned out that he was better at math when it was related to an avid interest than he had been in math class at school.) If so, it needs just as much enhancement as do these other more nontraditional pathways to success.

Key 4: Be a Safety Net, Unconditional Advocate, and Support System for Your Child

Easier said than done? A presumptuous pronouncement when *of course* this is the role you're trying to fill for your child? Maybe you had both these reactions to reading Key 4. We all want to do the absolute best for our children, and we all fall a bit short sometimes, especially when ADHD makes it a bigger challenge than it might be for other parents. Yet I emphasize this point here because sometimes friends, relatives, educators, or even professionals advise us to go against these parental instincts and engage in a "tough love" approach to the sometimes difficult behavior of teens or young adults with ADHD. That approach advises kicking them out of the house and otherwise abandoning them as if this will somehow make them "wake up and smell the coffee" and behave like typical peers. But that is a losing strategy in dealing with teens who have a neurodevelopmental disorder like ADHD. Being tough with them doesn't change the underlying neurological limitations that give rise to their difficulties with self-regulation. And you know in your heart it is wrong to abandon people with disabilities just because they don't act the way typical peers do. Please rest assured that the entire purpose of this book is to help you fill this role day after day, by using its 12 principles to guide your parenting.

I know how important this is, because in virtually every instance of success by the children with ADHD I have known, many of whom I've followed to adulthood, a key to their healthy adjustment and success was the fact that they had at least one parent or other loved one who never gave up on them. That person was always in their corner and never quit believing in them in terms of accepting the child for who he or she was and not what others wanted the child to be. Sometimes children with ADHD just need someone to be on *their* side and not just the side of conventionality, obedience, authority, righteousness, or decorum. This person should also be open to the nontraditional and unconventional routes to success illustrated in the examples above. Undoubtedly you're already that person. This book is intended to help you stay in that role.

In my experience, this parent or other relative or caregiver provided a support system for the child, and not just a financial one. More important was the emotional support system or "bank account" set up with the child, into which the parent made "deposits" of affection, approval, respect, encouragement, and other signs of love and support (in the words of Stephen Covey, author of *The 7 Habits of Highly Effective People*). To quote a divorce attorney describing the one thing he felt made marriages succeed or fail: *Love is a verb!* You have to do it frequently to have it and to get it from others. Daily kindnesses add up to create close and strong relationships. Making daily deposits into your child's emotional bank account gives you plenty of "savings" to help maintain your relationship when you have to make withdrawals (constructive criticism, etc.). And those credits make it more likely that your child will listen to your advice.

PRINCIPLE

2

REMEMBER THAT IT'S
A DISORDER!

Just as important as keeping your focus on the keys to success for your child (Principle 1) is reminding yourself that your child is dealing with a real disorder. Doing so buttresses your positive practical and emotional support with compassion, acceptance, and forgiveness. It also allows you to adjust your expectations in a way that will reduce family conflict and enable you to fulfill the child's greatest potential.

> **THE PROBLEM:** Your child looks as typical or normal as any other child, so it's easy to forget the child has a real disorder or disability.

In all of my decades of clinical practice and research related to ADHD, one of the greatest hindrances to helping those with the disorder has been the fact that other people, including parents and teachers, do not view it as a real condition. They view ADHD as a behavior problem that is the result of the child's willful choice to act this way or of bad parenting. Either way, it is viewed as a learned and likely voluntary behavior, probably used to get attention or escape from responsibilities. Therefore it warrants no compassion and in fact might deserve punishment. There is no reason to provide accommodations, protections, entitlements, special educational services, or anything else one might do for "real" disabilities like Down syndrome or cerebral palsy or for serious mental disorders like intellectual disability, psychosis, or autism. Harsh moral judgments and sanctions might be in order, but not compassion and a desire to be of help.

We can see why the public would hold such a view about ADHD: As I mentioned earlier, the very name trivializes the condition. Also, the disorder expresses itself through altered behavior and thus behavioral problems, which for far too long were attributed to poor parenting or teaching, or bad influences in the community. Finally, ADHD comes with no obvious physical signs that would tip anyone off to the fact that a child has a physical disorder or disability. The child or teen with ADHD looks as normal physically as any other person of the same age. The fact that such children and teens can do many things as well as typical peers conspires with their typical appearance to lead people to think there is nothing physically or neurologically wrong with them.

THE SOLUTION: Keep a disability perspective.

When I was starting my career in child clinical neuropsychology in the 1970s and working with children with developmental disabilities and neurological disorders, I came across the inspiring work of Dr. Leo Buscaglia, who promoted an uplifting view of life in general and an attitude toward disabilities specifically that were both quite inspiring. His book *The Disabled and Their Parents* gave sage advice to parents raising children with disabilities. And among the lessons in that book that has stayed with me in the 45 years since its publication was the importance of mindset in promoting a more helpful and humane way of understanding and assisting the disabled. His message was to acknowledge their condition yet treat them with dignity, have compassion not only for disabled children but also for their parents, and to embrace acceptance of their disability as just a part of the unique totality of that person. I have been teaching this principle to parents ever since.

We can't control everything that happens to us in life, but we can certainly control our attitude toward it. And as we know, attitude is everything in coping with adversity. This is also among the most insightful and even therapeutic lessons of Buddhist psychology. Life involves suffering; but how we react to suffering is what can bring further problems. Our attitude or interpretation of events will determine how we feel and respond, and these often involve wanting, longing for, or insisting on something different from what has actually happened to us. Acceptance of our reality can often relieve us of this additional suffering. Cognitive-behavioral therapy (CBT) makes the same key point. The disparity between what we want and think we should have or deserve and what is actually the case is the cause of our distress, depression, grief, anger, or anxiety. Our interpretation of events and not the actual events themselves is the origin of such unhappiness.

The fact that children with ADHD can act like typical youth conflicts significantly with the actual nature of their disorder. This disparity can throw you off in the midst of parenting, making you forget that your child can't behave like everyone else his age. You watch your son walk out of his room, leaving a disaster scene in his wake, and note how much he resembles his siblings in appearance and his friends in his demeanor in this particular moment in time. How easy it is to feel a flash of frustration that overall he doesn't *act* like them. Blame or criticism is just a short step from this emotional response.

This is a very natural reaction. Part of what we're responding to in such moments is grief—sadness that the child we love faces these challenges and so do we. Unfortunately, we humans sometimes reject sadness and turn to anger and blame instead. So these moments can be an important pivot point: With a disability perspective as our mindset, we can extend compassion instead of blame (and while we're at it, extend a little compassion to ourselves). Taking this fork in the road is much more likely to lead to strategic solutions that will help the child and us. (It's important not to get so focused on "solving the problem," however, that we start to try to reengineer our children and end up right back at not accepting them for who they are. See Principle 3.)

As the Introduction explained, ADHD is very much a real neurodevelopmental disorder that requires support and accommodations. Rather than merely an attention problem, ADHD is a developmental disorder of executive functioning and self-regulation that would more aptly be named executive function development disorder. Seeing how this takes shape as the problems you encounter with your child every day can make it much easier to remember that your child really can't help it—although he *can* be helped to do better and better over time.

Keep in mind, however, that the last thing a child with ADHD needs or wants is sympathy or pity. What children with ADHD want is your understanding—your knowing and accepting the fact that they may be different from you and their typical peers in several important abilities or capacities. Hopefully, your understanding and acceptance will cultivate compassion naturally. But even more important, it should create a willingness on your part to get them access to accommodations (see the box on the facing page) and treatments that can reduce the impairment from their disorder that occurs in certain settings and situations, such as school and even at home.

To me, this change in attitude or mental reframing of your child or teen with ADHD is brick one in building a treatment program. No other effective changes to that child's circumstances are likely to occur unless and until parents, teachers, and others accept ADHD as a real disorder that warrants compassion, accommodations, and other forms of treatment. It is the most important and essential change that has to happen as one begins the process of understanding ADHD in a child or teen.

As a parent who chose to pick up this book, you already understand that your child has a disorder; that's why you're reading this volume. Yet it's easy to forget in the most challenging moments of your day with your child. In general, it helps to:

- Renew your understanding of ADHD as a disability and thus

- Recharge the batteries of your compassion for your child and

- Recommit to undertake whatever accommodations and treatments the child may require in order to

- Reduce the impairments that arise from that disability.

I know that's a pretty broad directive; read on for specifics.

THE PROBLEM: Your child's neurodevelopment lags behind that of children without ADHD.

Decades ago, when I was about 10 years into my clinical work and research studies on ADHD, I thought it would be interesting to try to determine just how delayed children with ADHD might be in their executive abilities and self-control. I had already come to understand ADHD as a developmental disorder of self-regulation, and ADHD had long been thought to involve a developmental delay in attention, inhibition, and managing activity levels. So I looked across many different studies of children of different ages, including my own research, and computed just how deficient

Defining Our Terms

We are tossing around a lot of terms here, so let me be clear about what they mean.

Disorder: As I mentioned earlier in this book, a mental *disorder* is a failure or dysfunction in a mental capacity or suite of mental abilities that all humans possess. It can result in a significant degree of ineffective functioning in major domains of life activities. When that ineffective functioning reaches a point where adverse consequences begin to occur (the environment starts kicking back), a person is considered to be impaired by the disorder.

Symptoms: *Symptoms* of a disorder are the cognitive and behavioral expressions of that disorder.

Impairments: *Impairments* are the adverse consequences that occur as a result of those symptoms leading to ineffective functioning.

Disability or handicap: Impairment in functioning in a specific domain of activity—such as employment, education, mobility, or self-care—that results in harm or adverse consequences is a *disability* or *handicap.* Notice here that a handicap or disability results from an interaction between the limited capacity of the individual (the disorder) and the demands of a particular setting involving a major life activity, such as one's job. The handicap from one's disorder may be reduced merely by altering the situation. If the setting is changed, known as an *accommodation,* the person may be less impaired or even unimpaired by the disorder in a given circumstance. For example, putting a ramp at the front entrance to a building in no way eliminates the physical disorder a person may have that hinders her mobility and confines her to a wheelchair. But it does reduce the disability or handicap in that situation—she can enter buildings that previously were inaccessible to her. In that situation, she is disordered but not handicapped or disabled.

children with ADHD were on various measures compared to healthy control children.

The 30% Rule

As I mentioned in the Introduction, brain scans have shown that children and teens with ADHD are on average a few years behind others in their executive brain development. My research years ago and my reading of others' research showed that the range of executive function deficits was somewhere between 22 and 41% of what typical children were able to do on these tasks, averaging about 31%. This was just an initial effort to get some idea clinically of how far behind in development children with ADHD might be in their executive functioning and self-control on average, but out of it came the highly useful idea that children with ADHD seem to be, on average, about 30% behind healthy typical children of the same age.

What does the 30% rule imply for how we should understand and support children with ADHD?

1. *We cannot expect children with ADHD to function at the same level as typical children in their seven executive abilities and in their self-control.* They simply can't do so on a routine basis.

2. *A great deal of the conflict between the child with ADHD and others was rooted in the inappropriate expectations that parents, teachers, and other adults had for such children and teens.* A clash was occurring between what was being demanded of the child and what the child could actually do on his own given his ADHD. So instead of thinking or saying, "Why can't you act like other children?" we should be thinking or saying, "What can I do to help you do what other children are able to do on their own?"

> **THE SOLUTION:** Adjust your expectations to your child's executive age.

Simply put, *lower your expectations for your child's ability to regulate behavior and then think about what accommodations you could make so your child can succeed despite executive function deficits.* Not only will doing so evoke more compassion in you regarding your child's inability to do what others her age can do, but this solution leads to important practical strategies.

If we take the chronological age (CA) of the child with ADHD and reduce it by 30%, we can get a rough idea of what the child's developmental level is in executive functioning—I call this the child's *executive age* (or EA). So, EA = CA × .70 (70%). It's not meant to be rocket science, demanding great precision—just a rough idea of where your child may be functioning. That means the average 10-year-old with ADHD may be functioning more like a 7-year-old in self-control. And that is about what we can expect from the same child in his day-to-day functioning when it comes to self-awareness, impulse control, attention span, working memory, emotional control, self-motivation, time management, and self-organization/problem solving. Your child *can* do these things; just not at the level other children are able to do them.

For instance, your child is 10 years old, in fourth grade, and has been given a typical amount of homework for someone in fourth grade, say 40 minutes. Is this reasonable given the 30% rule? No, not even close. The amount of homework and the degree to which we expect the child to do it independent of assistance from others should be like what we expect of a 7-year-old: 5–10 minutes. What can you do about this? For one thing, get the teacher to reduce the amount of work the child has to do for homework. That will help, but the child may fall behind other children in academic knowledge and skill if this sort of adjustment goes on for a while. She would not be doing as many problems as others and so perhaps not becoming as proficient at this task or concept as others. Alternatively, break up the assignment into smaller quotas more consistent with the child's EA of 7 years. So, give her 5 minutes' worth of work to do, then let her take a break for a minute or two, then give her another 5 minutes of work to do, then another short break, and so on until all the work is done. Will all this take longer than it would for another child? Yes. But not as long as it now takes for the child with ADHD to get the work done on her own (she won't get it done anyway). And at least it will get done, and with a lot less stress, conflict, and tears than if you had just told her to go do her homework like you might a typical 10-year-old.

One more example of how thinking in terms of EA changes expectations: Your son with ADHD is 16 years old, which means in the United States he can probably get a driver's license. Should he? No! Not for independent driving. Why? The 30% rule tells you why. You just gave someone with the self-control of an 11-year-old a car. OMG! What were you thinking when you did that?

This teen needs to perhaps delay even applying for a license. If he does apply, he needs to stay at the learner's permit level longer, practicing under adult supervision. Then as he demonstrates greater ability to drive with you in the daytime, you might let him drive with you at night. Then eventually he can drive alone. If that goes well, maybe he can have one friend in the car. Notice that you give him only as much independence as he shows he can handle. If he doesn't handle that next level of independence well, you drop back to the earlier, more supervised level.

Related to this issue is the teen's problem with being distractible and having little impulse control. Knowing that, should he be allowed to have a smartphone in the car while driving? No, not without some constraints on its use. You can't just tell him not to use it. We know that given his lower EA he won't abide by that rule once driving alone. You have to make using it while driving impossible. How? By downloading an app into the phone that prevents it from being used while the car is moving. Or by installing an inexpensive device in the car (usually in the smart port somewhere on the dashboard) that will block all cell signals when the car is turned on. Again, the point here is not the specific advice for driving— it's the understanding that comes from knowing your teen has an EA that is much lower than his chronological age and adjusting your expectations and accommodations for him accordingly.

You can apply this 30% rule to just about every major demand you may be making on your child with ADHD, especially as new opportunities for independence come along for her (dating, driving, part-time work, managing money, going to college, etc.). What changes would you have to make in these activities for a child who is 30% younger than her age in self-control to be able to handle them well? It also forces you to consider if you should be letting your child or teen do these things at all right now. The most important thing to remember here is not the number (30%) or its scientific precision (it's not), but the simple yet profound fact that a child with ADHD is substantially delayed in their development of self-control and executive functioning. Now armed with that fact, use it to adjust your expectations downward as if your child were functioning at a younger developmental level (EA) in their daily life activities.

> **THE PROBLEM:** Your child's disability can be frustrating.

I don't have to make a case for this claim; you're living it. So, in those moments when your patience is exhausted and so are you, it can be easy to think "I get that you're disabled and I can handle what that entails most of the time, but *this*—THIS—is just too much. I know you can do better than this!" When patience runs out, compassion can be hard to come by. So let's try another tack.

> **THE SOLUTION:** Practice forgiveness.

I'll show you what this might look like in the conclusion to this book, where I help you put all the principles together to use them in parenting your child with ADHD. Hopefully it will suffice here to say that forgiveness can be a good practice when the bar for misbehavior seems to have been raised, or a consequence of your child's symptoms feels more devastating than usual. Sometimes the best response is to forgive your cherished child for what really isn't his fault anyway and simply move on. This advice is woven throughout the principles in the rest of the book.

With an understanding that your child has a disorder, and with acceptance and compassion, the tactical benefit of applying the 30% rule, and forgiveness in the most trying moments, you'll have:

- ▪ Far less conflict in your parent–child relationship
- ▪ A far greater likelihood that you will make all the necessary accommodations and engage in the most appropriate treatments
- ▪ A much greater willingness to advocate for the child in getting appropriate medical, educational, and psychological services
- ▪ A much greater likelihood of promoting your child's development, adaptive functioning, and general welfare

So don't let the brevity of this chapter fool you—viewing ADHD from a disability or disorder perspective is among the most important principles in this book.

3

BE A SHEPHERD,
NOT AN ENGINEER

If you read Principles 1 and 2, you're already getting a sense of what this principle is all about: that as parents we are shepherds, guarding our children, keeping them safe, promoting their welfare, and helping them do the best they can with the strengths and weaknesses they have. The keys to success in Principle 1 include being there unconditionally for your child and seeking out the best supports in your community, and the theme of Principle 2 was compassionate acceptance in the midst of realism. I only wish the entire parenting population was on the same page.

> **THE PROBLEM:** Parents as engineers or architects.

Nearly everywhere we turn these days, we are inundated with advice about how to raise our children. Just now, I searched Amazon books for titles that dealt with "raising children" and was immediately informed that more than 80,000 were available. You can bet they all do not agree with each other. This is a recipe for parenting paralysis. There was even one book called *Raising Children for Dummies,* as if you could learn how to expertly fashion a child just as you would learn to operate a computer or repair a car. If only there were a website like *ConsumerReports.org* or *Edmunds.com* where you could just go and search out all the makes, models, styles, and options for a child as we do when buying a car. Just specify everything we want and be told just where, how, and how much to pay to get it. We could even get feedback on the average results to expect in our community.

From all this you would think that parents are largely uninformed when it comes to how to raise children—that we have no natural inclinations about how to bring up our children to be healthy, well-adjusted, well-adapted, and contented adults. Yet plenty of children survived—and thrived—well before the 19th and 20th centuries, when a whole new class of experts arose to advise us on how to raise children (and wrote lots and lots of articles and books about it). The emergence of an entire industry surrounding parenting also implies that somewhere there must be a blueprint we can count on, if only we could identify that single best schematic. And, finally, the natural conclusion to draw is that if all these instruction manuals are out there, it must mean that children are a blank slate at birth and that we parents have incredible powers that we can use to design them. We can determine what they will be like, what sort of personality they will have, how intelligent they are and will become, and how successful, accomplished, and happy they will eventually be as adults. All this could lead us to believe that we start out as novice parents but can actually become skilled architects and engineers of children.

Can We Design Our Children?

How did we get to this point? Undoubtedly a number of forces combined to convince us today that we can (and should) become practically perfect parents and end up with optimal children who turn into model adults. With the many astounding advances the last century or so has seen in technology, science, and information delivery, it's not surprising that we've come to believe in our powers of innovation and problem solving. We've also seen trends in parenting advice come and go and, because we're so devoted to our children, tried to adopt the recommendations of the experts of the day. It's all well and good to try to learn how to promote children's healthy growth and development and to be the best parents we can be. The problem is that along the way many of us have forgotten how to trust our intuition, to rely on our intimate knowledge of our children, and have ended up believing not only that it is possible to craft a better child if we can only identify the most authoritative expert, but that if we fail to do so and our children are not well behaved, successful, and happy, it is our fault.

From the standpoint of biology, evolution, genetics, and the entire span of human history on Earth, this is largely utter nonsense. Of course, parenting matters. A lot. But maybe not in the ways you think. And we parents certainly don't have the power to redesign our children and shouldn't burden ourselves with guilt for failing at such engineering efforts. But it's a tough treadmill to get off these days with all the pressure we experience to be perfect parents. If you have experienced any of the items in the box on the facing page, then you likely have gotten stuck on that treadmill and might want to consider getting off it now by shifting your mindset.

Your Rusty Inner Guidance System

Far too often we ignore our own instincts and our intimate knowledge of our own children because we are deluged with parenting advice, devalue much of the wisdom previous generations have passed down, and forget how diverse children are even when raised by the same parents. There are no designer children—there never have been, and cannot be! Yes, we need to study child rearing scientifically to glean what we can about even better ways of raising our children to the extent that is possible. But that should not result in the unquestioned belief that children are blank slates and we alone get to determine the course of their lives. Parents are not architects, engineers, or chefs. Parenting isn't cooking!

Believing that we can engineer a perfect child is particularly damaging to parents whose children are born with any one of myriad (more than 250 at last count) developmental, psychological, or psychiatric disorders that may emerge during that child's development. Most often it induces tremendous guilt over the role the parent may have played in raising an imperfect child. Furthermore, it produces tremendous grieving over what might have been but now seems lost—the perfect, capable, and well-adjusted child we so craved who was within our reach had we only relied on the current science of parenting. See the box on pages 47–48 for a summary of the evidence that we cannot engineer our children.

The Take-Home Message

Your parenting does not matter as much as you may think. Don't get me wrong: Parenting certainly does matter. No one is telling you to abandon your children or "just leave them a loaf of bread and go to Las Vegas," as one

Do You Need a Parenting Reality Check?

Many of us have unrealistic expectations of what we can achieve for our children by being good parents—and end up feeling disappointed and guilty when the outcome isn't perfect. If you experience any of the following, you can benefit from Principle 3.

❑ Are you overwhelmed with parenting advice? Paralyzed because of it? Bewildered by all the contradictions in it?

❑ Are you afraid to act or not act in certain ways toward your children because of what parenting experts have said or written?

❑ Do you believe that every interaction you have with your child has a lasting impact? That the approach you take to child rearing is critically important?

❑ Is your sense of parenting competence so low or fragile that you are afraid others are critical of your parenting when you are out in public with your children?

❑ Do you think that your child's entire fate is in your hands? Has this made you an around-the-clock parenting machine?

❑ Do you find yourself hovering over your child whenever you can do so to manage everything he thinks, says, and does?

❑ Do you try to prevent your child from experiencing any distress, frustration, or failure for fear it may warp her mind, personality, or behavior for life?

❑ Have you sacrificed your marriage, your personal interests, or your leisure time with friends to parenting?

❑ Do you worry that making your children unhappy with you will warp them for life and that they will require long-term psychotherapy to recover?

❑ Do you believe your child's ADHD is your fault even though you have read the scientific evidence that it is a biological, mostly genetic neurodevelopmental disorder?

(continued)

> If you checked a lot of these boxes, you're hardly alone. This parenting mindset is one reason we worry so much about whether we're doing right by our kids: everyone else seems to be doing it, so if we're not, aren't we abdicating our parental responsibility? And when we have a child with a disorder like ADHD, these worries are magnified. Although it might feel hard to do, you'll find that relaxing a bit more in your parenting will do both you and your child a world of good.

parent comically accused me of implying. But it matters in ways that are different from what we have been led to believe. Certainly, our myriad daily interactions with our children matter; they are very important in determining the relationship we will have with our children for the rest of our lives. So long as your child is adequately protected, clothed, nourished, guided, and stimulated, you will have provided a good enough environment inside your home for him to blossom, develop, and even flourish.

But other decisions you will be making as to what is outside your home are far more influential than what you may do inside it. Those decisions have to do with where you choose to live, what kind of neighborhood surrounds your home, what other children your child will be exposed to, the quality of the schools the child will attend and the teachers who will attend to him, the other adults in that community with whom your child may have contact, and the resources available to you to enhance your child's natural abilities and aptitudes. These are the ways that parents mainly influence the psychological nature of their children—indirectly, by arranging for good environments around them. Remember, it is the unique environment that your child experiences that is not shared with their other siblings and that is largely outside your home that matters more here. Research in child development repeatedly shows that unique out-of-home experiences and settings along with genetic predisposition seem to matter far more to your child's psychological development when compared to the way you deal with him inside the home, short of parental neglect, abuse, or child malnutrition. So long as parents provide a "good enough" environment for a child, the more important influences are outside the home.

So, if you do not matter as an architect or engineer of your children via your child rearing, how do you matter?

How We Know Perfect Parenting and Perfect Children Are a Myth

Still not convinced? If you find yourself wringing your hands over your failings as a parent of a child with ADHD, take a look through this list of reasons we know that your power is, well, not that powerful.

■ *Premodern children.* If the modern view of parenting as all-powerful is accurate, how did so many past generations of children ever survive, adapt, and succeed, and how did their parents raise them to maturity, without parenting books by experts?

■ *Siblings.* Whether you look at your own siblings, your children, or your friends' families, it's impossible to deny the marked differences among those raised by the same parents. In most cases, parents do not radically alter their parenting for each and every child they raise. It's the children's own inherent differences and characteristics that have more likely risen to the surface.

■ *Identical twins.* Why are identical twins raised apart since birth by entirely different parents highly similar in so many ways—not just in appearance, but in intelligence, personality, talents, interests, preferences, psychological characteristics, psychiatric disorders, and even gestures? Yes, we can find some small differences, but they are minor and certainly less numerous than are the similarities. Yet they were raised by entirely different parents and undoubtedly parented in entirely different ways than was their twin. If parenting is so powerful, why are they so similar?

■ *Adoptees.* All of the research on adoptees who have been raised by unrelated parents since birth shows one striking finding— the personality, intelligence, mental abilities, psychological characteristics, psychiatric disorders, and many other attributes of these children are significantly correlated with those of their biological parents and not at all with those of the parents who raised them. Yes, they may attend different churches or be in different political parties from their biological parents, but other than such differences due to social influence, why don't these children more closely resemble their adopted parents?

(continued)

■ *The research evidence.* Large studies that have followed children across their development, including large numbers of identical and nonidentical twins, have revealed that:

Genetic differences are a major component of the differences among children.

The influence of parenting (shared environment) is always less than that of genetic influences.

Over the course of development there is a marked decline in the degree of parental influence, which is greatest in the preschool years and becomes virtually nonexistent by late adolescence or young adulthood.

Nonshared, out-of-home environments account for individual differences to a significant degree.

The influence of those out-of-home effects increases with age across development and exceeds that of parenting by or before adolescence.

Genetic influences on specific traits may increase over development.

■ *Causes of children's psychological and psychiatric disorders.* We now have massive evidence that most disorders are the result of neurological and genetic effects and not due to parenting or shared family environment. (See the fourth edition of *Taking Charge of ADHD,* for details.)

■ *Rates of mental disorders in children.* Finally, why are rates of children's psychological and psychiatric disorders either remaining stable or increasing if the science of parenting has improved so substantially? If we knew so much more about parenting now and parenting caused these disorders, then those rates would decrease, and they haven't.

THE SOLUTION: Be a shepherd, not an engineer.

Your child is a unique being. Every one of us has a unique mix of strengths and weaknesses in (among other traits) the seven executive functions. That means that you get the chance to shepherd that unique person into adulthood by understanding where each executive function is most and least developed in your child and providing supports accordingly to help her become the best-developed and most effective person possible. But you do so indirectly and primarily through the pastures in which you choose to raise the child and the resources you provide. You are not a sculptor to the child's clay, but a guide, supervisor, provider, nurturer, protector, sponsor, and all-around shepherd to what is and will be a unique individual. Understand your part here and you can more easily impart essential things to your child, all the while enjoying this developmental show as it plays out. You get to play the important role of shepherd—you don't get to design the sheep!

What to Do?

So, what do good shepherds do? They certainly don't desert their flock and head to the nearest bar.

1. Provide protection. Good shepherds keep watch over their sheep day and night and ensure that the harms of the world are much less likely to befall them. Job one of any parent is obviously protection of their child from the nefarious forces at play in our homes, neighborhoods, schools, and larger communities. So you do what parents instinctively do: search out and eliminate as many sources of harm as you can, monitor your children, and see that they get the most appropriate care and treatment when needed to cope with and hopefully recover from such harms. Children with ADHD are three to five times more likely than other children to experience accidental injuries and poisonings; to experience bullying, victimization, and physical and emotional abuse at the hands of other children and adults; and to generally get into more trouble because of their penchant for risk taking and sensation seeking. They are also nearly twice as likely to die from an accidental injury before age 10. Most parents are psychologically wired to engage in this protective behavior instinctively.

But these protective efforts are especially important for parents of children with ADHD.

2. Do whatever you can to find the best neighborhood in which to raise your child. I don't mean to be insensitive to the fact that not all of us have a lot of choices here, but often we have some discretion. Does your neighborhood provide good-quality schools, other good shepherd families, prosocial peers, other adults who can be good role models, and other resources that can foster your child's physical and social development, like sports, clubs, scouts, and church groups? As Judith Harris said in her book *The Nurture Assumption,* where you choose to buy or rent a home has more to do with your child's development than what you are likely to do inside of it. Find the best neighborhood that you can reasonably afford. Then monitor your child's relationships and steer the child toward developing relationships with prosocial, psychologically well-adjusted, and even inspiring peers. In doing so, don't forget the increasingly important role of the Internet and social media and monitor your child's time online too.

Encourage your child with ADHD to play a lot, get physical exercise, even participate in scheduled routine exercise activities at a health club or in organized sports. Physical exercise is especially beneficial for children with ADHD because it seems to help reduce their symptoms and improve their emotional health and self-motivation, and it helps them cope better with the difficulties they encounter. It also contributes to maintaining appropriate weight (obesity can be a problem for children with ADHD) and overall health and wellness.

3. The younger your child, the more your interactions matter. I noted earlier that this does matter with the youngest kids, and it matters to your ongoing relationship.

Creating predictable, supportive, rewarding, and stimulating interactions with your child does initially help him become better adjusted and more confident and competent. Make your home life, rules, routines, family rituals, and other recurring activities reasonably predictable, and as pleasant and respectful as you can. Keep your interactions with your child stable, supportive, rewarding, respectful, and predictable, not chaotic, emotional, capricious, or disparaging, and don't be psychologically absent or uninvolved with them. A good number of the principles that follow in this book are designed to do just this—provide a predictable, rewarding, approving, accepting, loving, and nurturing shepherd and pasture.

4. Make adjustments as needed to accommodate your child's limitations. We will discuss many specific accommodations you can make in particular circumstances and for certain tasks later in this book. The point here is that you can reduce how handicapping a condition is by changing the environment so your child is less impaired in a given situation. For instance, you might have your child do her English homework at the kitchen table while you are preparing dinner, set a timer for completing a small quota of problems (such as three to five problems, as I suggested earlier), allow short breaks from work, dispense encouragement and approval throughout, touch her lightly but affectionately on the shoulder occasionally as a further sign of approval, or reward her with her choice of dessert after dinner. Doing so in no way changes your child's degree of ADHD. But it does make it much more likely that your child will complete the assignment than had you given her all the work to do at one sitting with no break, in her bedroom, unsupervised.

5. Look for any ways you can to improve your child's settings to make them more educational, stimulating, or just fun to be in and interact with. Adding a swing set to the backyard, more books in the bedroom for nighttime reading, more educational toys, DVDs, constructive educational video games, and more sports gear to the home environment can have a positive impact on a child's development.

6. Provide good nourishment. Take a close look at your child's diet and overall nutrition to see if it is contributing to current and longer-term health and wellness. Or is it excessively slanted toward junk, starchy, sugar-laden foods and beverages? On average, children with ADHD eat less nutritiously than typical children. We think that is because those foods are what your impulsive child with ADHD gravitates toward and will make less of a fuss about eating. And that has led to marked risk for obesity among children with ADHD that increases with age as does the risk for type 2 diabetes. By adulthood, twice as many people with ADHD are clinically obese as are typical people. So, is it possible for you to provide access to more balanced and nutritious foods and reduce and remove the less nutritious ones from the house? Some children with ADHD have vitamin (usually D), omega 3 or 6, or iron deficiencies that could be best addressed through their diet. A small percentage may have allergies to food colorings that can worsen their symptoms of ADHD. Ask your pediatrician if this might be the case and what steps you could take to address these deficiencies and allergies.

7. Provide consistent and predictable settings and routines. Examine your own household routines to be sure you are making them as consistent and predictable from day to day as is feasible.

- Are the morning routines before school consistent and effective at getting children prepared and out the door for school?

- Are your dinnertime and evening routines also fairly consistent in when you eat, do homework, prepare your children's things for the next day, bathe or shower, brush their teeth, and get them off to bed?

The routines of families who have children with ADHD are often inconsistent and chaotic, leading to poorer eating, dental, medical, and sleep hygiene or consistent use of preventive health maintenance practices with their children. Such an unpredictable home environment increases stress in the family and especially on the child with ADHD, whose own coping abilities are impaired due to this disorder. Stress can make your child's ADHD worse and also sow the seeds for developing oppositional and defiant behavior. Sometimes this inconsistency is due to one parent also having ADHD, so be sure parents are properly evaluated and treated for ADHD and related conditions.

8. Take good care of yourself. You can't be your best at raising your child if you are experiencing significant health problems, emotional distress, or general life stress. So inventory your own life.

- How is *your* weight, nutrition, use of alcohol and any other substances you are prone to use excessively?

- Are *you* exercising enough to remain in reasonably healthy physical and mental shape?

- Are *you* getting enough sleep so you are not a fog-brained, irritable, emotionally brittle, or spaced-out shepherd?

- What are you doing to recharge your emotional batteries so you can better cope with and shepherd your child with ADHD?

Many parents find that routine exercise, sports activities with other adults, clubs, church groups, yoga and meditation classes, or immersion in their hobbies restores their emotional well-being. So make sure you don't skimp on emotional self-maintenance while dedicating yourself to being the best shepherd you can be for your child with ADHD.

If you have concentrated on improving those areas above that you found to be in need of attention, then you have done as much as you can to be a good shepherd to your child with ADHD. The rest is largely not within your power to control. You now get to raise a unique individual while trying to sustain a close and supportive relationship with your child across your lifetime. So having done your best, enjoy the show!

GET YOUR PRIORITIES STRAIGHT

Speaking of shepherds, taking care of even one child with ADHD can sometimes feel like herding cats. This is why it's so important to get a handle on what you really need to get done, whether it's keeping your child on schedule, enforcing house rules, or keeping up with household chores. In my work with families, I've found that the best-laid plans often prove flawed. We're all human, things happen, and before you know it your to-do list is as long in the evening as it was this morning. When it comes to what they expect of their child, I advise parents of children with ADHD to try to prioritize what will promote the child's development and functioning, and when it comes to managing home and family, to take into account what will reduce their own stress levels so they can keep going.

> **THE PROBLEM:** Parents of children and teens with ADHD often have arguments with their kids over minor issues, triggering increased family conflict.

Because of their ADHD symptoms and the broader problems they have with self-regulation and executive functioning, children and teens with ADHD have lots of difficulties following through on instructions, chores, school assignments, and other requests. This lack of compliance is frustrating to parents, who then typically repeat the command (possibly many times), getting increasingly angry as their child fails to start or finish the required task. If you're familiar with this sequence, you know that too often the result is an explosion over something that in hindsight may seem laughably trivial. Let's break down how this happens a little further:

Children with ADHD resist shifting away from an activity they're enjoying to comply with a request to do something else more than other kids. Even typical adults sometimes procrastinate at starting work when there are more appealing ways to spend their time. But those with ADHD, especially children, have a limited capacity for emotional self-control and less tolerance for waiting and delayed gratification. Their aggravation at being asked to do anything that isn't fun can easily lead to conflict with parents.

This defiance can evolve into oppositional defiant disorder (ODD) and escalate battles between children and their parents. Often within 2 years of developing ADHD symptoms, children develop ODD, which involves abnormally high levels of anger, hot-temperedness, hostility, arguing, defiance, noncompliance, stubbornness, irritability, and even vindictiveness. An important dimension in the development of ODD is the interactions between child and parent(s). This is not to say that the conflicts over unmet requests that are typical with ADHD directly cause ODD by themselves. But they can play a role in the development of ODD when coupled with the child's own limited emotional control, so it's always important to minimize such conflicts. One way to do that is to get your priorities straight.

The huge number of requests that all parents typically make of their children is really tough on kids with ADHD—and ineffective when the goal is to get things done that you believe need to get done. Researchers have found that parents may issue 100 or more different commands or instructions to their children *every day.* If we assume children are awake for about 15 hours a day, that's an average of at least six commands every hour, or one every 10 minutes. Even typical children may have trouble listening to them all, keeping track of what they're supposed to be doing, and following through. With their attention deficits, distractibility, and impulsiveness, to say nothing of hyperactivity (think of watching your 7-year-old try to sit still long enough to finish homework as you've instructed), children with ADHD will find this long list of dictates overwhelming. Now imagine how *any* 7-year-old might feel when Mom gets angry or disappointed when he doesn't get the homework done in the designated time frame because he really can't meet the demands of doing so. As this scene repeats day after day, his frustration builds, his sense of self-worth drops, and he gets angrier and angrier at Mom. The child begins to expect Mom's disapproval, Mom begins to expect a battle, and the potential for conflict mushrooms.

> **THE SOLUTION:** Reconsider priorities and change the dynamic.

There are a number of ways you can change the request–resistance pattern that feeds conflict.

1. Start by figuring out whether you can simply let some requests go, at least for the time being. Take a look at the different kinds of requests you and all parents tend to make of children:

■ Instructions to stop some behavior or another that you find annoying

■ Requests for the child's help in getting something done, such as a brief request to get something you need

■ Requests for more time-consuming help, such as with doing the laundry

■ Instructions to do the things children should be doing for themselves as part of learning their own self-care, health maintenance, and daily functioning (dressing, bathing, brushing teeth, eating properly, picking up their own messes, etc.)

■ Instructions about getting homework done

■ Instructions and reminders to do the household chores the child or teen has been assigned

Did you notice that some of these feel less essential than others? If your child just finished clearing the dinner table and taking out the garbage—especially without any argument—maybe this is not the time to ask him to run upstairs and bring you your iPad. Or if it's been a full day for your child (and you), the dishes and garbage can wait till the morning. The point is that keeping peace in the family and in your relationship with your child is always a high priority. There are some requests that are always going to be less necessary than others, and there are always moments when even something that is usually a high priority should drop down to prevent conflict.

2. Review the situations or times of day when you and your child seem to be particularly prone to conflict. When do you typically brace yourself for a fight with your child? Bedtime? Homework time? In the morning before school? It can be very revealing to pick one of these times of day that's usually problematic and write down what you ask of your child at that time. Let's say you find that this is what you expect (and verbally request) of your child before school:

- Wake up at a reasonable time to get ready for school

- Take any prescribed ADHD medication as soon as possible

- Use the toilet

- Get dressed

- Make the bed

- Put pajamas back in their drawer

- Put away any toys on the floor

- Put any dirty clothes in the hamper

- Brush teeth

- Put the cap on the toothpaste and put it in the medicine cabinet

- Wipe out the bathroom sink

- Hang wet towels on the towel rack

- Eat breakfast

- Put cereal bowl and juice glass in the dishwasher

- Have all necessary school materials in the backpack

- Put the backpack by the door

- Feed the pets

- Find and put on a coat (if it's cold weather)

- Get lunch money from parents (as needed)

- Leave for the school bus, walk to school, or get into the car on time

- Give Mom/Dad a kiss before leaving for the day

Pretty long list, eh? Maybe you need to return to Step 1 above. Is it really so important that your child make her bed before going to school, put her pajamas back in the chest of drawers, tidy up the bathroom, or put her dishes in the dishwasher? Is *all* of what you are requiring essential? And does all of it have to be done at that time? Could any of the things you're asking your child to do be deferred to a better time to engage her in this request?

3. Now ask yourself how you want this time of day or situation to end. As Stephen Covey said in his book *The 7 Habits of Highly Effective People,* you should begin this situation with the end in mind. How do you want the morning to end? You probably want your child to go off to school clean, dressed appropriately and comfortably, fueled for the day's learning, equipped with the necessary school materials, and supported by the knowledge that he's loved and appreciated by you. Here's what the list above would look like with these goals in mind:

- Wake up at a reasonable time
- Take ADHD medication (if necessary)
- Use the toilet
- Get dressed
- ~~Make the bed~~
- ~~Put pajamas back in their drawer~~
- ~~Put away any toys on the floor~~
- ~~Put any dirty clothes in the hamper~~
- Brush teeth
- ~~Put the cap on the toothpaste and put it in the medicine cabinet~~
- ~~Wipe out the bathroom sink~~
- ~~Hang wet towels on the towel rack~~
- Eat breakfast
- ~~Put cereal bowl and juice glass in the dishwasher~~
- Have all necessary school materials in the backpack
- ~~Put the backpack by the door~~
- Feed the pets

- Find and put on a coat (if it's cold weather)
- Get lunch money from parents (as needed)
- Leave for the school bus, walk to school, or get into the car on time
- ~~Give Mom/Dad a kiss before leaving parents for the day~~

You just eliminated 11 potential points of conflict! (You might argue with a few of these deletions, but note that as long as your child has packed his backpack, you can probably remind him to go get it from his room. And as to getting a kiss, it's more important that you offer one.) With the image of how you want the morning to end clearly in mind, you'll find yourself acting toward your child in ways that are more likely to achieve that end. Those will be very different from what you might have done had you not thought about this issue. (For further help, see references later in the chapter to other principles in this book.) Thinking with the end in mind also helps you focus on what is essential to get done in the upcoming morning routine. It also invites you to consider what you could easily let slide for the sake of getting the essentials done and doing so in the most peaceable and respectful way.

4. Ask yourself, "Will complying with this request help build my child's development and functioning?" In other words, who benefits from this request? You, your child, or both of you? Only directives that focus on the last two beneficiaries should be priorities for you right now. It might not be worth arguing over busy work, tasks your child can't begin to do yet due to executive function deficits, and things that would make your life easier but don't really build your child's self-awareness, competence, accountability, or ability to sustain attention. You might know that sticking to a schedule for walking the dog helps your son learn time management and accountability. But if he also has to do his homework and pack his equipment for baseball practice on time, perhaps the dog walk can wait or be assigned to another family member today—the other tasks on your child's agenda will already be helping build time management and accountability. Or let's say you have a house rule that all members of the family must hang up their bath towel and put all their dirty clothes in the hamper before leaving the house. Is enforcing this house rule important every day if your child with ADHD happens to be struggling to meet other requirements before leaving the house on this particular morning?

5. Ask yourself whether this command has to be obeyed right now. Maybe what you want your child to do is important, but is now the best time to ask that he do this task for you, or is it something that you have requested just because it came to mind and you hadn't really thought about the best time to do it? Keeping his bedroom relatively clean and organized may be of some small to moderate importance for your child and for you, but is a school morning the best time to make such a request? Isn't Saturday morning a better time, when there is no hard departure time for school and work to bump up against?

6. Figure out how important and how urgent it is that a particular request be met by your child. None of the preceding advice means you should never ask your child to do certain chores that involve straightening up the house. But it does mean leaving some of those requests to a stretch when there is more time to do them and for you to supervise them, and there is less pressure to meet a deadline for leaving the house, such as after school or on the weekend. In sum, you need to decide which battles to fight with your child over getting things done at a particular time and which, at least at that moment, are not worth fighting.

In the workplace, many people use the four-square method (or Eisenhower grid) as a simple way to understand their priorities. Pick a request that typically causes conflict and think of it as falling into one of the four boxes in the grid below.

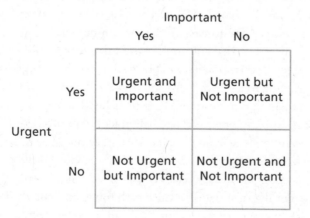

		Important	
		Yes	No
Urgent	Yes	Urgent and Important	Urgent but Not Important
	No	Not Urgent but Important	Not Urgent and Not Important

All too often, we get caught up in asking our children or teens to do the things that fall in the two boxes stacked in the right column. They are either **Urgent but Not Important** or neither of these (busy work). Their urgency can make it seem like they need to be done right away, so we tend to do them. But when examined more closely these activities may not be very important at all. These are the sorts of things you should consider letting go for a while and not asking your child or teen to do them. Asking your child to empty all the wastebaskets in the house just before bedtime can seem very urgent if you've just realized that the garbage pickup is tomorrow. But in most cases letting the trash remain unemptied till next week is not a tragedy in the larger framework of life. The request may not be very important or, as it turns out, very urgent. It can be put off until Saturday morning chores and ignored on that particular school night in favor of more important goals for your child (homework, family time) and for you (less conflict with the child, less stressful running around by you or anyone else).

An example of something **Not Urgent and Not Important** (lower right in the diagram) might be having your child make her bed before school. Making a bed has little or nothing to do with preparing to go to school. And it is not important as a priority in helping your child develop well. Yes, being reasonably neat and tidy and caring for one's room are nice things, but not essential. You may feel better when the house is all in good order, but could you let this aspect of household organization slide sometimes? Or, as I suggested above, could it wait until Saturday morning if you think it is important that your child do it for you or with you at least sometime during that week?

Now let's think about things that are **Urgent and Important.** As in business and other types of adult employment, these are the sorts of things we all do with little problem. Their urgency ensures they get our attention and, combined with their importance, clearly motivates us to tackle them ahead of other things. For instance, your child or teen may have a science project or book report due the next morning, so it becomes urgent that it be finished by bedtime that evening. And it is important because it will count as a major part of the child's grade. We ignore such projects at our children's peril. So they usually get done. On a school morning, having your child properly cleaned, dressed, fed, and organized for school as well as maintaining a positive and loving relationship with the child are the Urgent and Important things we do.

There are also things we want our children to do that are **Not Urgent but Important.** This is usually where parents need to focus more time and effort to help their child or teen develop properly, remain well adjusted, and be prepared for life. These might be any of the following:

- Respecting parents and other family members
- Getting along reasonably well with siblings
- Being honest in dealings with others (not lying)
- Making friends with other children
- Managing emotions properly, particularly in a social context (inhibiting aggression, moderating frustration)
- Participating in organized community activities (such as clubs, scouts, sports, or church groups)
- Respecting others' property and possessions both inside and outside the home
- Obeying laws
- Age-appropriate self-care (dressing, bathing, dental care)
- Accepting responsibility for one's actions and their consequences

These and other important domains of functioning in major life activities are rarely urgent. But they are incredibly important to a child's overall development and adjustment. Notice that I have rephrased unacceptable behavior (lying, fighting, stealing) into its more appropriate positive alternative. I do this so that you can focus on the behavior you want to encourage, approve, reward, and generally support in positive ways. Phrasing behavior in negative, unacceptable terms focuses your mindset and hence attention on punishment and other means of discouraging inappropriate behavior. We want to focus on rewards *before* punishments, encouraging prosocial behavior before acting to suppress its unwanted alternatives, if necessary. (See Principle 7.)

Whenever you find yourself considering requests that always seem to trigger arguments or defiance, ask yourself the following three questions:

- **"Does this have to be done** to promote my child's welfare?" [Is it Important?]
- "Does it have to be **done now**?" [Is it Urgent?]
- "Does it have to be done **by my child** now?" [Whose priority is it?]

If the answer to all three questions is yes, then have at it. But it usually isn't. I can't say that you'll immediately be able to tell the difference, though. We parents are only human, and when you've been involved in a lot of conflicts that seem pointless because "it would be so easy to do what I ask!," you might start to dig in your heels. But if you try to step back to get a little objective distance (the next principle can help), you might be able to see what's really urgent and important more clearly.

An Important Caveat

When determining what's urgent and important enough to ask of your child, you do have the right to consider your own well-being. Keeping your home picture-perfect at all times probably shouldn't be a top priority—especially above the healthy development of your child and the welfare of the whole family—but if being surrounded by a mess makes it impossible for you to concentrate on going about your day, you can undoubtedly find a comfortable middle ground. Maybe asking your child to make his bed in the morning feels like a way to contain the chaos in which you feel you're living, and excessive stress does affect how able you are to be there to shepherd your child (see Principle 3) effectively. But perhaps there's another way: What feels more stressful, leaving the bed unmade or making it yourself sometimes? The point is that only you can make the decisions that are right for your child with ADHD, for you, and for the family as a whole. I've found over and over again, however, that flexibility and compromise are critical to setting priorities that serve everyone best.

7. If you're having trouble getting your priorities straight, consider a family meeting (or family counseling). Sometimes conflict really takes hold of a family and it feels impossible to step back and get enough distance to reset priorities. When that's the case, why not call a family meeting? Ask everyone to review the conflicts that are arising and how they could be prevented. This discussion alone might lead, more quickly than you think, to a consensus on how various requests can be moved up or down on the list of priorities. But if this doesn't seem practical, or you try it and the meeting just erupts into more conflict, consider getting some professional help (see the Resources).

If you do opt for the family meeting, be sure to stay on the topic of the meeting and not get sidetracked into other issues that aren't relevant or previous disagreements that you feel have not been fully resolved. Stay on task. To that end, follow this six-step procedure:

■ Define the problem as specifically as you can and even write it down at the top of a sheet of paper.

■ Invite all participating family members to come up with any suggestions they have for dealing with this problem. Give free rein to even far-fetched, impractical ideas besides those that are most obvious.

■ Do not engage in any criticism during this solution generation discussion.

■ After the list seems to be a good one with various ideas on it, go back and ask what each family member thinks of particular solutions. If there are three family members, then each gets to say "plus" for "I like it," "minus" for "I don't like it," or "zero" or "N" for feeling neutral about it—the person could live with that solution and doesn't feel strongly one way or the other about it. Mark that symbol next to each potential solution (+, −, 0) for each family member in the discussion.

■ After this brief evaluation period, look down the list for the solution that most people could agree with or felt neutral about. Choose that one, circle it, and make that the plan to try over the next week. If it is helpful, have each family member put his or her initial on this page to indicate having agreed to follow that solution for now.

■ After 1–2 weeks, call another family meeting to review how well that initial solution has helped to address that problem. Make revisions to the plan as needed. Then try it again for another 1–2 weeks.

Is There an Upside to Living in the Now (Ignoring Time)?

The answer is "Sometimes, but not all the time." Just as we understand that having a chronic problem sensing and managing time can be disastrous (see the Introduction), we can also appreciate that being obsessed with time, time management, and preparing for the future generally can also be problematic, not to mention highly stressful. You want your child to get chores and other tasks done on time, but again, it's important to consider priorities.

An excessive preoccupation with getting ready and getting things done on time can lead to passing up enjoyment of the moment. When setting priorities for both yourself and your child with ADHD, keep this in mind. The pleasure in life is often in appreciating the now and getting out of our own heads and our own way. Why do you think mindfulness, meditation, yoga, Buddhism, and alcohol and marijuana use are so popular? By various means, they all serve to telescope time back down to the now or the moment and the fabric of the reality around us. It's also why we go on vacation—to get off the treadmill of time management.

Because people with ADHD are more involved in and attentive to the now and not the future, we seem to find that they have far less trouble and may even be at an advantage in a crisis. By definition, crises are unplanned and unanticipated. They require that we deal with problems that are happening right now and make quick decisions about them. People with ADHD may not be at a disadvantage in situations that place a premium on dealing with the now and doing so decisively rather than contemplating the future and how best to plan for it. Physicians and soldiers with ADHD have told me that they did as well as or better than their peers when dealing with crises in the emergency room or in battle.

Children with ADHD live in the now and pay attention to it more than others, while giving less consideration to the future. While I want you to help your child with ADHD pay more attention to time, the future, and getting work done on time, the goal should be a good balance between paying attention to time, the future, projects, assignments, and deadlines, and remaining connected to and appreciative of the now.

8. If a request you want to make meets the three-question test, try using other principles in this book to pose the request effectively:

■ Be proactive (for example, set up a transition plan before starting this activity) (Principle 12).

■ Make your child or teen more accountable (more frequent and closer supervision while the child is working and with immediate consequences) (Principle 6).

■ Keep your instructions to a minimum and deliver them personally (touch more, talk less) (Principle 7).

■ Make the task or situation more rewarding or motivating for the child by offering some incentive and following up compliance with praise and rewards (Principle 7).

MINDFUL PARENTING

Be There and Be Aware

We all know how easy it is to be with our children but not really *be* with them at all in any sense of being attentive or even sociable. Even when they're right next to us, we're on our phones or tablets, immersed in e-mail and social media. Or we're somewhere else in our heads, preoccupied with work we need to get done tomorrow and goals we need to reach next week or next year—or ruminating over what happened yesterday or last month that could have gone differently. In the last chapter I made the point that it's a mistake to become slaves to time, and yet we all do it, because there never seems to be enough of it.

> **THE PROBLEM:** Parents are too mentally preoccupied when with their children, missing opportunities to promote better behavior and a better relationship with them.

All of these demands for your time and mind can easily distract you from what is usually one of the things you value most in your life—your children. And when your child has ADHD, your relationship is already at risk due to the stress and conflict created by trying to get through daily routines successfully. Principle 4 suggested ways to get out of the negative loop of constant demands that can threaten your relationship with your child. Here I help you take these efforts one big step further, giving you ways to prevent your time, attention, and emotions from being hijacked, so that you can invest them in creating and maintaining a close relationship with your child that will continue through both of your lives.

A good shepherd has to be attentive. A good parent has to be with and enjoy her child, just for who the child is. A good parent of a child with ADHD has to try harder to pay attention to the positive to appreciate both her child and herself.

THE SOLUTION: Become a mindful, attentive parent.

> Nothing is more humbling, more challenging and more heartbreaking than parenting. There is no quitting and no hiding and no "finish line." Therefore, as an act of self-preservation, we must actively cultivate kindness and compassion in the moment, mostly for ourselves.

Those words from Lisa Kring, a licensed social worker who teaches mindfulness, are doubly true for parenting a child with a neurodevelopmental disorder like ADHD. The stresses and challenges of doing so are magnified by the greater difficulties such children will pose, the delays in their development, the misunderstandings the public has about parenting such children, and the greater need to engage professionals and their treatments in the service of these children. Add in the possibility that you or another one of your children has ADHD, and the hurdles become harder to overcome. What can you do about it? Stop allowing your thoughts and emotions, ruminations, distractions, smart technology, and social media to hijack you away from your relationship with your child or teen with ADHD. How do you do that? Cultivate mindfulness.

Mindfulness enhances well-being. Mindfulness and the practice of mindfulness meditation have swept through our culture in recent decades for good reason, as an attitude, mindset, or stance toward living in our world and especially in dealing with others. The skills and perspective that mindfulness teaches have been shown repeatedly in research to:

■ Reduce stress in people's lives

■ Improve their quality of life

■ Allow them to cope better with sources of suffering including chronic illness, pain, and impending death

■ Help them attain more contentment, if not happiness, with their life circumstances

■ Contribute to better relationships with others

Mindfulness helps us appreciate the reality of life around us. Mindfulness promotes getting out of your mental preoccupations, ruminations, and future (goal-directed) thinking and being more aware of the moment and your surroundings. All of these forms of distracted thought command your attention and take you away from the reality that surrounds you right now. When you stop to pay attention, you notice that where you are in this moment is pretty wondrous and miraculous, much more than your environment may seem when all you're focused on is the mundane responsibilities and frustrations you have to deal with. Mindfulness teaches us that periodically letting go of our goal-directed thinking and our minds' general propensity for wandering and instead focusing our senses and attention more generally on what is present in this moment can endow us with more appreciation of our life and others, more peace with ourselves and with others, and a greater sense of unity with life and the world.

Mindfulness encourages us to appreciate what exists around us, especially our children. *Don't just be there; really BE with them in that moment and in that place.*

Mindfulness helps us cast off the "woulds" and "shoulds" that only make us miserable. Many people think of mindfulness, especially meditation, as a Buddhist practice, but you don't have to adopt any religious beliefs to develop and practice mindfulness. In fact, to me mindfulness is a valuable form of CBT, the treatment that helps us change our thoughts and behavior to change how we feel. Mindfulness shows us that when we intentionally stop overthinking things and stop being so inwardly preoccupied, we jettison our "woulds" and "shoulds," as cognitive behavioral therapists call them—the thoughts we have about the way the world ought to be or we wish it to be instead of the world around us as it is. It is this mental rumination and longing for what we want and often cannot have that is the basis for much of our suffering in life. That is an essential principle of CBT and not just of mindfulness (or Buddhism). Our thoughts and their associated emotions often are our own worst enemies and greatest sources of distress. When you're constantly focused on how your child with ADHD *should* behave or what you *should* do to keep your household running, you can't see the uniquely lovable child before you or enjoy the wonder of being that child's parent.

Mindfulness gives us a sense of belonging to something larger than ourselves. By getting out of our head, mindfulness teaches us to sense and value the totality of the immediate moment and our surroundings, including the fact that we are part of it rather than separate, as our preoccupation with our mental lives can often make us feel. A recent study showed that the greater happiness, or more accurately, sense of contentment, often attributed to religious individuals is actually not a result of their religion. It stems from this sense of oneness with reality and our universe that cuts across the religious, the nonreligious, and the atheistic or humanistic. By promoting a sense of belonging to something larger than ourselves and being an integral part of all life and the universe, we can achieve the same degree of contentment. We can have compassion for ourselves, as Lisa Kring suggests, and for our child, as integral parts of the world we exist in at this moment and every moment.

So, the main route I recommend for being there and being aware is to practice a secular form of mindfulness, especially when you're with your child, and perhaps even meditation. It's a great way to reduce parenting stress, achieve some degree of contentment with your life as it is, to appreciate, attend to, and even approve of your child as she is (and not as you want her to be), and so to build a more peaceful and lasting relationship with your child.

Through mindful parenting, you can come to recognize your own thoughts, emotions, and emotional triggers and replace automatic reactions to them—those knee-jerk responses that you may regret—with mindful actions. But more important is that you become more aware of, attentive to, and appreciative of your child not just for his good behavior but for his very existence in your life. Especially if you feel your relationship with your child is suffering, mindful parenting may be the best solution.

To make a new habit of being there and being aware, I encourage you to employ mindfulness in four ways:

1. Practice being mindful when you're by yourself as one would do while meditating. Think of these periods as practice drills, like those you'd do to improve at a sport or other skill.

2. Extend this type of mindfulness to special play times with your child or times of interaction with your teen using a method developed more than 40 years ago by Constance Hanf, PhD, a mentor of mine, which I have taught to thousands of parents as part of my behavioral parent training program.

3. Extend this type of interaction with your child to his independent play. Periodically find your child and briefly be mindful of, attentive to, and appreciative of—even in small ways—whatever it is the child is doing that you find positive, prosocial, or satisfactory.

4. Extend this pattern of mindful parenting to episodes when your child or teen is complying with your requests or performing other tasks.

As Jon Kabat-Zinn put it so nicely in an interview regarding his book on mindful parenting entitled *Everyday Blessings*:

> Mindful parenting is a lifelong practice. It means you become less attached to outcomes and more mindful of what's unfolding in your life and your children's lives. Mindful parenting is about moment-to-moment, open-hearted and nonjudgmental attention. It's about seeing our children as they are, not as we want them to be. We let everything that unfolds in life be the curriculum for our parenting—because it is—whether we like it or not.

Practicing Mindfulness Alone: Meditation Drills

The purpose here is to have you practice what it means to be mindful or fully in the moment and aware of all your senses while trying not to think too much and letting your mind be more fully aware of yourself and your surroundings. It's better to do this initially with your eyes closed. Vision is our dominant sense, and the things we see around us can trigger chains of thinking that distract us from being in, attentive to, and even appreciative of that moment. That's why people close their eyes when they meditate, I think. It's far easier to be master of your senses and thus your mind when the dominant sense is shut down or at least restricted initially. So, for 15–20 minutes daily at least four times per week, set aside time to be alone somewhere in a relatively quiet, distraction-free setting. This can be anywhere that you can be alone for 15 minutes. I have done this at work in my office, while at conference centers where I could find an unused room, in my car while waiting to pick up my grandson from school, and of course at home. "Wherever you go, there you are," to quote the title of one of Jon Kabat-Zinn's popular books. So find some private space and do the following:

Adopt a **sitting or reclining** position (don't lie down; you might fall asleep).

Close your eyes (gently relax your eyelids; don't close them tight).

Take a **deep cleansing breath** and then exhale slowly. Do it another one or two times if you find it helps you relax. Then just breathe slowly, regularly, and naturally as you might when falling asleep. But don't sleep.

Perform a body scan. First, do a muscle tension scan, as I like to think of it. You start with your head and neck and focus on relaxing the muscles in these areas. I find it helps to move them back and forth a little by rocking from side to side a bit. Or tense those muscles and then let them relax if that helps to relieve any tension. Then work your way down your body parts and major muscle groups (shoulders, arms, chest, abdomen, legs, and feet). Then do a body sensory scan. Again, start with your head, neck, and face and focus on what you are feeling or sensing in that area of your body at that time. Pressure, heat, contact with things like clothing or the chair surface? Just focus on it. If you feel some tension, try to relax those muscles again. Again, proceed down your body, simply attending to what you sense in each region. I do these two exercises because it starts my mindfulness meditation period by helping me to stop thinking and start attending to my sensory impressions.

Perform a situation scan. This is like a body sensory scan except now you are scanning your surroundings with your senses (except vision) for what you hear or otherwise sense. The point here is to just become more aware of it. Is a clock ticking? Can you hear an aquarium motor or refrigerator running? Can you hear your HVAC system blowing, or traffic, birds, or other sounds just outside? Just note them and move on.

Choose an attention focus for your mind; then concentrate on it. You are going from scanning your body and surroundings to a slightly more difficult drill, focusing your senses and mind on one recurring thing. Usually it's your breathing or heartbeat, but it can be anything within you or outside of you (ticking clock, repetitive sounds) that you find easy to attend to and return to if your mind wanders, which it most undoubtedly will. I sometimes close my eyes and focus on my breathing initially. Then I shift to what to me feels like staring at a point in the farthest distance ahead even though my eyes are closed. I am looking into that void as if something in the distance will appear in my mental imagery. You don't need to do that if it feels foreign or weird to you. Just find an attention focal point that you can concentrate on with your mind. You can create one if you like just by humming to yourself very quietly or even just in your mind.

Avoid thinking about anything. Stay on your focal point as much as possible. Surely all minds want to wander in this state. Yours will too. So, if thoughts occur, don't worry about them. Just note them, acknowledge their arrival in your mind, then bid them goodbye and let them go. Now get back to your attention focus. Don't dwell on the thoughts, pursue them, interpret, or judge them in any way. Just note that they happened and then release them like a butterfly and return to your attention focus point.

Be aware of sensations while attending to your focal point. While I am attending to my focus point, I also find I have a heightened sense of other things, like the contact I have with things around me, with sounds, and even with my internal states. Just like the occasional thought, I take notice of them and then move on to my focal point again. This heightened sense of surroundings is part of being mindful of them. Many people feel that this is what makes them sense that they are part of and integrated with their surroundings and even the larger universe. It's as if you are one thread woven into the fabric of that moment in reality. Most people find this to be a very peaceful and contented feeling. They are bathed in their sense of that moment and their surroundings.

Stay in this flow of moments and "nows" for about 15 minutes or more, then open your eyes. Stay put. This is sort of like waking up from sleep. Just become visually aware of what is around you. Continue your relaxed breathing and just notice all the things around you. Let your eyes roam about your entire visual field, taking it all in. I like to pay attention to the colors, textures, spatial arrangements, and other features of the things that surround me in the room, including patterns of light and shading, much like an artist who would be painting this scene might do. Again, try to let any thoughts that arise go uncontemplated and just release them to fly away. Try to stay in this moment for a few minutes.

Then slowly stand up and get back to your usual activities. Notice that you will do so with a heightened sense of things around you and of being more in the now and mindful of yourself and your context.

Throughout the day, practice mindful minutes. Just take a minute from time to time throughout your day and stop your thinking so as to just sense, feel, and attend to that very moment. You are trying to bring about states of mindfulness of moments on demand, whenever you need them. And you will need them when you are with your child or teen with ADHD. So just practice being in that moment and setting for that minute or two, then get on with your day. I'd recommend you try these mindfulness practice drills for a few days before moving on to the next exercise.

When you feel stressed, use the S–T–O–P method:

1. **S**top what you are doing. Build in a brief pause to allow yourself the time to become more aware of yourself and your surrounds.

2. **T**ake a breath. Breathe in slowly, deeply, and then exhale slowly. Do this several times to help calm yourself.

3. **O**bserve. Take in yourself, your surroundings, and what may be happening around you more fully—what is happening inside you, outside you, around you right now.

4. **P**roceed. With this mindful pause, you are far more likely to choose a more adaptive, effective, and genuine action as you proceed to deal with the situation—one that promotes your longer-term welfare and your relationship with your child or teen with ADHD.

How long should you do this before moving on to the practice described in the next section? We all differ in how quickly we pick up on this mindful state of mind. You decide when you're ready.

Practicing Mindfulness of Your Child during Special Playtimes: Paying Attention to Good Behavior

Hopefully the practice drills have shown that you can easily slip into a state of mindfulness whenever you have a few minutes. And while practicing meditation with your eyes closed can help you enter this state of being totally aware of the now, the point of those practice drills was to help you learn to do this with your eyes wide open.

This child-focused playtime involves setting aside 15–20 minutes each day as a special time to play with, attend to, approve of, acknowledge, appreciate, and otherwise be mindful of your child as she is at that moment. This is both valuable practice and a good investment. As a practice it prepares you for the later exercises of paying attention to your child throughout the day, especially when the child is complying with your requests. It's an investment in that it will improve your relationship with your child and thus pay you back for the time you've put in. Everyone wants to feel appreciated. When children sense that they're appreciated, they have more respect for those who attend to them and are often more willing to listen to, comply with, and generally be more helpful toward such people.

I've found that doing these play exercises four or five times a week helps parents focus on and appreciate the behavior and good qualities that the child usually displays during these special playtimes. And it's not complicated. You surely know that people who are rated as the best managers, the best team members, and the best friends and partners are those who seem to be more attentive to and appreciative of us when they're with us. When we feel unappreciated, we often change jobs, quit teams, divorce our partners, and end friendships. Your child can come to feel the same way if all you do is bark orders or argue with him and ignore him when he's behaving reasonably well—such as when you're caught up with your social media or brooding about the future. The box on pages 76–77 gives step-by-step instructions for paying attention to your child during special playtimes.

Practicing Mindful Attending to Your Child throughout the Day

Once you feel confident that you can be mindful in special playtimes with your child, move on to being mindful throughout the day. Especially with a child who has ADHD, parents tend to "let sleeping dogs lie"—ignoring the child who's not being disruptive and seems occupied. It's understandable to use this time to get other things done, but you may be missing numerous opportunities to encourage such independent behavior by essentially ignoring it. Especially if you instead pay attention to your child

Paying Attention to Your Child's Good Play Behavior

Paying attention to your child's play behavior involves the following:

1. If your child is under age 9, select a time each day as your "special time" with your child—after your other children are off to school in the morning if you have a preschool child or after school or dinner if your child is of school age or you work outside your home. No other children should be involved. Set aside 15–20 minutes each. If your child is 9 years or older, just find a time each day when your child seems to be enjoying a play activity alone. Stop what you're doing and begin to join in the child's play, following the instructions below.

2. For a younger child: At the designated time, say, "It's now our special time to play together. What would you like to do?" For an older child, ask if you can join in on whatever your child is doing. Let your child choose the activity—no TV. Otherwise, don't take control.

3. Relax and casually join in. Don't start this playtime when you're upset, busy, or about to leave.

4. After watching your child's play, begin to narrate it, showing enthusiasm to convey to your child that you find his play interesting. Think of yourself as a sportscaster. Young children really enjoy this. With older children, you should still comment about their play, but less so.

5. Ask no questions and give no commands! This is critical. Avoid questioning the child except to clarify how your child is playing if you're uncertain of what she is doing. Give no commands or directions and don't try to teach the child.

6. Occasionally provide your child with positive expressions of praise and approval, or positive feedback about his play. Be accurate and honest, not excessively flattering. For instance, "I like it when we play quietly like this," "I really enjoy our special time together," or "Look at how nicely you have made that. . . . "

7. If your child begins to misbehave, simply turn away and look elsewhere for a few moments. If the misbehavior continues, tell your child that the special playtime is over and leave the room. Tell your child you'll play with her later when she can behave nicely. If the child becomes extremely disruptive, destructive, or abusive during play, discipline the child as you would normally do.

SUGGESTIONS FOR GIVING POSITIVE FEEDBACK AND APPROVAL TO YOUR CHILD

Nonverbal Signs of Approval

Hug
Pat on the head or shoulder
Affectionate rubbing of hair
Placing your arm around the child
Smiling
A light kiss
Giving a "thumbs-up" sign
A wink

Verbal Approval

"I like it when you. . . . "
"It's nice when you. . . . "
"You sure are a big boy/girl for. . . . "
"That was terrific the way you. . . . "
"Great job!"
"Nice going!"
"Terrific!"
"Super!"
"Fantastic!"
"My, you sure act grown up when you. . . . "
"You know, 6 months ago you couldn't do that as well as you can now—you're really growing up fast!"
"Beautiful!"
"Wow!"
"Wait until I tell your mom/dad how nicely you. . . . "
"What a nice thing to do. . . . "
"You did that all by yourself, way to go."
"Just for behaving so well, you and I will. . . . "
"I am very proud of you when you. . . . "
"I always enjoy it when we . . . like this."

Note. Adapted from my book *Defiant Children, Third Edition.* Copyright © 2013 The Guilford Press.

only when the child misbehaves, you're inadvertently teaching the child that misbehaving is the best way to get your attention. So do the opposite. Look for times when your child is doing something independently from you but near enough to you to go find him. Then go find him and briefly notice what he's doing and acknowledge, approve of, and appreciate it—working or playing well independently while leaving you to get other things done.

This takes only a few minutes, but it's not easy to remember to do it frequently. Try setting the timer on your smartphone, kitchen oven or microwave, or just an old spring-loaded cooking timer to chime every 20–30 minutes. Then when the timer sounds, go find your child and if she's well behaved, attend to and appreciate it. Creating a situation where your child has to behave well to earn this attention is described in the box on the facing page.

Practicing Mindfulness When Your Child Is Complying with Requests

Once you've gotten used to mindfully attending to your child while you're playing with your child in special time or when working on a task or chore independent of the child, you can start to practice being mindfully attentive and appreciative when your child complies with your requests. The box on page 80 explains how.

Though mindfulness parenting is not easy and takes practice, it is something to be incorporated into the way you live with and interact with your child or teen with ADHD as much as you can. The benefits of doing so will come back to you in many ways that are well worth your expending the time and effort to learn this approach to parenting a child or teen with a neurodevelopmental disorder.

Being Mindful of and Attending to Independent Play

Many parents complain that they can't talk on the phone, cook dinner, visit with a neighbor, and so forth, without the child interrupting what they're doing. The following steps were designed to help you teach your child to play independently of you when you must be busy with some other activity.

1. When you're about to become occupied with a phone call, reading, fixing dinner, and so forth, give your child a direct command that (a) tells the child what he is to be doing while you are busy and (b) specifically tells the child not to interrupt or bother you—for instance, "Mom has to talk on the phone, so I want you to stay in this room and watch TV and don't bother me."

2. Then as you begin your activity, stop what you're doing after a moment, go to the child, and praise the child for staying away and not interrupting. Remind the child to stay with the assigned task and not to bother you. Return to what you were doing.

3. Then wait a few moments longer before returning to the child and again praising him for not bothering you. Return to your activity, wait a little longer, and again praise the child.

4. Over time, gradually reduce how often you praise the child for not bothering you while increasing the length of time you can stay at your own task—praise the child every 5 minutes and then increase it to 10 and then 15 minutes.

5. If it sounds like your child is about to come bother you, immediately stop what you're doing, go to the child, praise him for not interrupting you, and redirect him to stay with the task you gave him.

6. As soon as you finish what you're doing, go and provide special praise to your child for letting you complete your task. You may even periodically give your child a small privilege or reward for having left you alone while you worked on your project.

Note. Adapted from my book *Defiant Children, Third Edition.* Copyright © 2013 The Guilford Press.

Being Mindful and Approving When Your Child Is Compliant

Now, when you give a command, give the child immediate feedback for how well he is doing. Don't just walk away, but stay and attend and comment positively.

1. As soon as you've given a command or request and your child begins to comply, praise the child for complying, using phrases such as the following:

"I like it when you do as I ask."

"It's nice when you do as I say."

"Thanks for doing what Mom/Dad asked."

"Look at how nicely (quickly, neatly, etc.) you are doing that. . . . "

"Good boy/girl for. . . . "

2. If you must, you can now leave for a few moments, but be sure to return frequently to praise your child's compliance.

3. If your child or teen does a job or chore without being specifically told to do so, provide especially positive praise or even a small privilege, which will help the child remember and follow household rules without always being told to do so.

4. Begin to use positive attention to your child or teen for virtually every command. Make a special effort to praise and attend to your child for complying with two or three commands that the child usually follows only inconsistently.

Note. Adapted from my book *Defiant Children, Third Edition.* Copyright © 2013 The Guilford Press.

PROMOTE YOUR CHILD'S
SELF-AWARENESS
AND ACCOUNTABILITY

If you've started to apply the mindfulness strategies from Principle 5, you're using your own attentive appreciation to encourage the behavior you want to see from your child. You're probably also reaping the benefits in a closer, warmer relationship between the two of you. With your new skills, you're now prepared to help your child take on some of the task of monitoring his own behavior, encouraging himself to keep up the good work and holding himself accountable when things aren't going so well.

> **THE PROBLEM:** Children with ADHD don't monitor their own behavior and are not very aware of themselves.

As you know from the Introduction, one of the executive function weaknesses in children with ADHD is their limited ability to monitor themselves, also known as self-awareness. Associated with that problem is one of diminished accountability to themselves and others for their actions. After all, if you're not aware of what you're doing and, especially, doing wrong, it's difficult to accept responsibility for your own actions or acknowledge that your behavior may warrant certain consequences. Depending on the context, "self-awareness" can mean different things, but here I mean the process of being tuned in to our ongoing behavior and feelings and knowing how appropriate they are for the situation and the pursuit of our goals.

The ability to monitor our own actions is important to functioning well in all of the arenas of life. Children who aren't aware of what they're doing and what they should be doing struggle to succeed because they don't always know whether they are:

▪ Behaving the way they wanted to in the situation they're in

▪ Adhering to appropriate social norms for conduct in that setting

▪ Performing a task or interacting with others in ways that will get them to their goals in that situation

▪ Doing well in getting to those goals

▪ Acting in ways that are adaptive and effective in promoting their longer-term welfare

▪ Behaving in ways that show that they both acknowledge and accept responsibility for their actions

Maybe you've seen your child functioning without the benefit of these aspects of self-awareness. You may have wanted to ask "What were you thinking?" several times a day. The answer is that your child wasn't thinking at all about what he was doing or its consequences. It's as if the mirror in the brain that we often hold up to ourselves for critical self-examination is smaller or warped in children with ADHD.

As Amanda Morin notes on the website *Understood.org,* self-awareness in children should promote self-evaluation and includes not only acknowledging their own actions but also:

▪ Recognizing their own strengths and weaknesses

▪ Identifying what needs to be done to complete a task

▪ Recognizing errors in schoolwork and making edits or changes

▪ Understanding and talking about their feelings

▪ Recognizing the needs and feelings of other people

▪ Seeing how their own behavior affects others

When researchers question people with ADHD about their behavior, they often show that they're not as aware as others of how well or how poorly they are acting or performing. And both children and adults with

ADHD often report that they perform better or are as competent as others in tasks or domains of life where they are actually doing more poorly than others, such as in their school performance, friendships, and driving abilities. It's not hard to see how these distortions in self-perception could cause problems for those with ADHD, and casual observation tells us that these deficits do cause children (and adults) with ADHD a lot of trouble. But little research has been done about the impact of weak self-awareness, and even less on how to promote this capacity for self-reflection and self-monitoring. Therefore, the solutions that follow are based largely on a combination of common sense and what we know from interventions for other disorders that involve weak self-awareness.

> **THE SOLUTION:** Use methods and tools for reviewing behavior throughout the child's day.

Consider the following strategies a toolbox and choose the methods and tools that you feel might work best for your child at his or her age. It's difficult for research studies to evaluate the internal workings of the mind, such as whether a child is monitoring herself at the moment, but it's possible to measure whether the task at hand has been accomplished, and on that basis all these methods show some success when used by parents and teachers.

Modeling and Coaching Self-Awareness

As for virtually all the other principles in this book, you are the best teacher your child could ever have.

   1. Set a good example. A very simple way to begin teaching your child to be more self-aware is to model this regularly. Think of this as performing a postmortem of the kind you've probably done often after an event where your effectiveness was important. Evaluate out loud how you did in a particular situation—what you did, how well it went, what mistakes you think you made, and then what you think you could do better next time. If other people were involved, talk about their feelings and reactions to what happened too. You can do this with situations at work or home or even social gatherings like parties you threw. You might do it after a parent–teacher conference or a consultation with your lawyer or financial adviser or doctor. If you look for opportunities to do this modeling, you'll not only show your child how to do such a self-analysis and how it can lead to ideas for improving behavior but also send the message that it's safe and normal to do so, with no loss to one's self-concept or self-esteem.

2. Narrate a social scene. Another method, this one recommended by the *New York Times*'s Learning Network, is to teach your child social self-evaluation by having her sit with you and watch a social situation involving other children, such as at a park or playground or shopping mall. You can both pretend to be TV reporters and narrate the behavior of the children you're watching as if it's a news event. You can guess at what might be going on, how one child might feel given what another one has done, and what each of you would do if you were involved in that interaction. Also report on the behaviors, facial expressions, or other things, like tone of voice, you might be noticing and whether they were appropriate or inappropriate.

3. Interview your child. Another way to introduce self-awareness to your child is to gently and kindly interview her about herself. Start with easy questions—"How tall are you?" and "What color is your hair?"— then move into abilities and activities: "How well do you do at soccer?" "Are you good at making friends?" "Do you get along with your brother?" You can get your child thinking about her strengths and weaknesses just by asking what her best subject at school is or whether she's better at drawing or running. You can also ask about feelings, such as how your child felt during a recent situation when she seemed embarrassed, giddy, frustrated, or angry. Don't interrogate your child but instead express curiosity and interest. When you ask these questions, you're modeling for your child the self-evaluative questions she can ask herself. Adopt a sort of thinking-out-loud, softer approach to asking these questions.

Random "Stop, Look, and Listen" Checks

One of the easiest and most common ways to help people self-monitor in situations is to randomly cue them to attend to their behavior and how they are doing relative to some goal or standard. For instance, if we were at a dinner party and my wife thought my voice was too loud (it can be) or the topic was controversial (often), then she might kick my shin under the table as a cue for me to monitor myself. I'm not suggesting here that you kick your child to encourage self-awareness, just that we can all benefit from occasional cues to stop and attend to what we're doing.

1. Use random timing and substantial consequences for not monitoring. Let's say you want people to be more aware of driving at or under the speed limit. In that case you could cue them to look at their speedometer more often while driving. Some states do this by putting up road signs that warn drivers that their speed is being monitored. But over time people get so used to these static cues that they lose their impact. It's important that cues be infrequent—randomly timed—and that the consequences for ignoring the cue be substantial. A surefire way to get drivers to monitor their speed is to put police cars or speed-sensitive cameras along roadways at unexpected times and places where people are prone to speeding. With your child, it's best to start by randomly cueing him to stop and examine what he's doing and how well it conforms to a rule or a goal. You can then add consequences to make your child more likely to do this on his own and to learn from it.

2. Use a timer to remind you to give cues. Try doing this self-review spot check randomly when you're with your child. You can just ask "What's up?" as a starting cue. The hard part here is not so much the cue you choose but for you to remember to do this. You can use the alarm function, stopwatch, or other timing device on your smartphone to remind you. Or try a timer on an oven or microwave or an old-school simple spring-loaded cooking timer. Just set it to go off at various intervals in some random order. You could set the timer for 5 minutes, then 20, then 10, then 3, then 25, and so on. Whenever the alarm sounds, that is your cue to go to your child and prompt him to do a "What's up?" or "Stop, look, and listen" check. Teach him that when you say, "OK, it's time to stop, look, and listen," he should stop, think about what he was just doing, tell you about it, and evaluate how well he's behaving in that situation. If your child had a task to do, he should tell you how far along he thinks he is toward completing the task and if his progress is good or too slow.

3. Consider picture cues. In classrooms for children with ADHD or autism, teachers or aides have used picture cues, sometimes taped onto tongue depressors or popsicle sticks with pictures of a small stop sign, big eyes, and big ears pasted on the ends of these sticks. The teacher simply holds it up, waving it back and forth a bit in the visual field of a particular child to cue her to stop and monitor what she's doing. Obviously teachers are most likely to do this when a child is not paying attention to what she's supposed to be doing. You can try this at home as well. Just get these pictures off the Internet or simply draw them yourself and paste those images on sticks that you can flash at your child while she's doing some activity. This sort of nonverbal cueing might come in handy when your child is doing homework or a chore, when she has a friend over to play, or when she's doing any activity and things sound like they're deteriorating. But you don't want to just do this cueing when the child is inattentive, noncompliant, or becoming disruptive. You also want to do such random spot checks for self-monitoring even when she's attentive, well behaved, compliant, and otherwise getting along with others. You are promoting self-awareness in general, not just awareness of bad behavior specifically.

The Turtle Technique

When I was supervising classrooms for kindergartners with ADHD in a public school years ago, we taught children that whenever we said the word *turtle* to them they were supposed to act like a surprised turtle—pull in their arms and legs to their sides, slowly move their head to scan the situation—and then, unlike a turtle, ask themselves what they were supposed to be doing at that time. Then they were to tell the teacher what they should have been doing. After that, they were to "come out of their shell," so to speak, and get on with doing what they were told to do. While teachers tended to use this method more when children were not complying with directions, we also encouraged its use even when children were well behaved. Again, we did so to promote general self-awareness of their behavior and not just awareness of misbehavior. Children who successfully acted like a turtle when cued to do so were given a little washable ink stamp on the back of their hand that resembled a turtle. Later in the day they could count up their turtle stamps and cash them in for play with special toys we kept in the classroom. Poker chips or other tokens could be used just as well as a rubber stamp. Again, this is also a method that parents could use to promote self-monitoring at home in young children with ADHD.

The Mirror Method

Years ago, I came across a research study of children with ADHD that examined how well those children might improve in their desk work at school if one were to simply have them do their work while facing a mirror. Remarkably, the children showed significant increases in the amount of work they were able to do with no additional intervention by the teacher. Think about whether doing something like this might help your child be more self-aware while doing her homework or another chore in a relatively small space with room for a mirror.

Another option is to prop up a tablet or smartphone in front of the child with the camera on and reversed so that your child can see himself on the screen while working. Of course, this comes with the risk of tempting the child to play a game on the screen instead of working, but even a mirror affords the chance to make funny faces at himself, so experiment to see if either approach helps.

Discreet Cues for Older Kids

Older children and teens may not want peers to see them being cued verbally, so researchers have come up with some nonverbal ways of cueing children that can be used not only in classrooms but also elsewhere when others are around.

1. The paper clip cue. For teens who tended to go off task or violate classroom rules, we worked with teachers to walk around fiddling with a paper clip, which they would then discreetly drop near the teen as a cue to get back on task. Other objects besides a paper clip can be used, as long as the teen is told in advance what the object signals. At home, one parent I knew used a particular card from a deck of playing cards to cue his son to get back to what he was supposed to be doing.

2. The random tone recording. One year very early in my career I was involved in designing and running a classroom for children with ADHD who were between ages 8 and 10 years. To teach them to become more aware of what they were doing when they were supposed to be working at their desk, we made a tape of a random series of bells ringing. The bell might ring in 15 seconds, then 2 minutes later, then 5 seconds later, then in 3 minutes, then in 30 seconds, and so on (like the random appearance of police cars to remind drivers to monitor their speed). When the bell rang, the children were to stop and ask themselves if they were doing the work they had been assigned to do. If so, they put a checkmark in the plus (+) column on an index card. If not, they put a check in the minus (−) column. At the end of the task or activity, they subtracted any minuses from the total of their pluses to earn points they could redeem later in the day for special playtime, use of special toys, or little snacks. With teachers scanning the room to make sure the students didn't cheat, the system worked beautifully at getting children to complete over 95% of their desk work on time despite having ADHD and being so distractible. And the children seemed to be much more aware of themselves while they were doing their desk work and would even mutter things to themselves about how they needed to stay focused on their work if they wanted to get the maximum number of points. You could use the same system for homework, a chore, or playing appropriately with a sibling.

3. The vibrating cueing system. Similar to the random tone cueing system, a company has developed a product called the MotivAider to use brief vibrating sensations rather than audible rings or tones. This small square device is worn on a belt or placed in a shirt pocket or attached to some other piece of clothing. The device has a digital timer visible on the front of it and buttons that can be used to set the timer to vibrate at any desired interval, say every 3 or 5 minutes. When the device vibrates, the child is to check whether she is doing as asked. There is also a button to push that makes the device vibrate at random intervals. Used by itself in this way, the device is simply a means to cue self-monitoring. But it can also be part of a reward system, just like the tone tape. When the device vibrates, if the child was working, she records a point on a card. Naturally, this is a harder reward program to supervise because a parent or teacher may not know when the device vibrates. So some trust is required of the child or teen to follow the rules of the reward program. Otherwise, the device works fine as just a nonverbal cueing system without rewards.

Children as Their Own Models

This is a method for improving self-awareness that I first became aware of in research on treatments for the social deficits and other problems associated with autism spectrum disorder (ASD). It has been found to work well in improving the social behavior of children with the disorder. Not only are they fascinated with seeing themselves in a smartphone recording of them playing with other children, but they can remember the review of it later, any comments about what they did so well with others, and any suggestions of what they could have done differently if a problem arose in the interaction. Although it is used to promote social skills in a child with ASD, I see no reason why this technique could not be used for this purpose in children or teens with ADHD. You may find that the next time you are in the situation where you used this technique, your child is more likely to remember that she played with other children and to know how to interact better with them. And I think it also has a broader application as a method for promoting self-awareness in particular problem situations even if the issue is not problematic social behavior with peers. The child or teen could be recorded for a few minutes at any time of day while working, involved in some chore or other task, playing with siblings, doing homework from school, or, yes, interacting with peers as was originally done for children with ASD. The method goes something like this.

When you're in a situation where your child may benefit from some feedback from you about his behavior or social skills, use your smartphone to record a video for a few minutes. Try not to be too obtrusive or obvious, but you don't necessarily have to be secretive about it either. Then, as soon as possible after that situation has ended, show your child the video and talk about the behavior recorded. Start with what the child was doing that was positive and appropriate. Then discuss what the child (and you) see in the recording that could stand some improvement. Talk with the child about what he could have done differently to behave better in that situation.

Bedtime "Day in Review" Sessions

Parents have been using bedtime to review the day with children for ages, and you can use this daily ritual to promote your child's self-awareness by going over what went well and not so well for her. It's important to avoid using this time to list the child's misdemeanors; keep it light in tone. Try starting with a review of your own day (modeling, as above) and then lead your child through her own review of her day. Young children may need gentle prompts if they can't seem to remember what major activities they did that day; older kids and teens may do better completing a journal about what happened, what went well, what went poorly, and how any problems can be handled better next time around.

Teaching Children Mindfulness Meditation

In Principle 5, I encouraged you to learn mindfulness to become more aware of your interactions with your child. Your child can benefit from mindfulness too. More than a decade ago, Susan Smalley, PhD, then a research scientist at UCLA, conducted a pilot study in which children with ADHD were taught mindfulness and its related practice of meditation to reduce their ADHD symptoms. She reported some encouraging positive results. But the study was flawed in various ways, so it did not offer definitive proof that children or teens with ADHD might benefit from this treatment. Subsequent studies have tried teaching mindfulness to children with ADHD with mixed results, finding that parents reported improvements in the child's behavior and, especially, compliance with instructions while teachers, who were not involved in the treatment program, did not notice any changes. Better results were obtained with teens with ADHD, in which case teachers did notice improvements in ADHD symptoms. But again, as recent reviews have emphasized, the research is not very rigorous, so more well-designed studies are needed to determine how well this technique may work. Even so, some parents have reported that their children seemed to gain self-awareness by participating in classes that taught mindfulness and meditation. So if such classes are available near you, and you think your child might benefit from them, there is little harm in enrolling your child. They may even offer your child a set of skills to use for her own stress management and emotional self-regulation, as they can for you (see Principle 5). Several books in print help parents teach mindfulness to their children or teens (see the Resources), and at least one book, *I Am at Peace: A Book of Mindfulness* by Susan Verde and Peter Reynolds, is meant for children themselves.

> **THE PROBLEM:** Children can't persist for long without being held accountable.

Children with ADHD have problems getting things done or behaving as instructed because they're simply not paying attention to what they're doing. The self-monitoring strategies above can help many of these children become more aware of themselves and their behavior and in turn enjoy more success at school and elsewhere. But self-awareness is only step one in this process. Step two is holding themselves accountable for their actions and accomplishments (or lack of them).

As discussed in the Introduction, executive function deficits make it hard for children with ADHD to work independently of others, to motivate themselves to sustain their work-related behavior over time, to follow through on rules, promises, and commitments, or even to remember what they have agreed to or been told to do by others. Long-term projects and time delays make it even more difficult for children with ADHD to follow through on their own on time. In addition, these kids find it hard to take responsibility for their actions. Because of their impulsiveness, they are more likely to quickly deflect responsibility by blaming others for what went wrong or why they misbehaved. They may even lie about their conduct and whether they did anything wrong in the first place.

For all of these reasons, children with ADHD must be held accountable to others more often than typical youth of their age if they are to become more self-aware, get things done, and behave responsibly. They can eventually learn to do this better on their own. But at first, they need your help. And you'll find the effort pays off. Simply installing some aids to keep your child accountable can eliminate lots of conflict and recriminations and make life easier for both of you. And you'll be working together instead of at odds, which is the kind of relationship we all want with our children.

THE SOLUTION: Hold them more accountable more often.

Being accountable means being responsible for your actions, for the things you agree to do, for following the rules in a situation or the directions you have been given, and for managing your emotions properly. Obviously, when you help your child improve self-awareness with the help of the strategies in the first part of this chapter, you provide a foundation for her to learn to hold herself accountable for her own actions. You're shepherding her toward a successful adulthood.

Make a Habit of Accountability Check-Ins

You can increase the accountability of children with ADHD in a number of ways besides working on self-monitoring. An obvious one is to check in on them or otherwise supervise them more often while they're supposed to be doing something they were assigned or agreed to do. Here are the components of an effective check-in:

- Ask the child to tell you what he's doing, even if you've witnessed it.

- Provide encouragement, praise, and other forms of approval and positive feedback for not only how much work the child has gotten done so far but just for reporting on what he's doing honestly. If you wish, also provide small rewards for the work completed so far.

- Tell the child that you know he can get this done.

- Say you will check back in again shortly to see what he is doing and how things are going. We're all more likely to follow through on a commitment when we know we're going to be held accountable for doing it by others.

What's important in these check-ins is that you are using positive-language questions to prompt self-awareness and self-accountability. There's a critical difference between this kind of talking and simply talking to get your child to obey some instruction, which I encourage you to do a lot less (see Principle 7). The following are some tips that parents have found useful for making check-ins most effective:

1. Break the tasks down into much smaller quotas of work than other children might be able to do alone. So instead of giving your child, say, 25 math problems to do, give him just five for now and either check on him frequently or have him let you know when he's finished those five. Then you can provide approval, praise, or even a reward for the work before assigning him five more to do, and so on. Each time you simply assign a relatively brief and easy-to-accomplish goal along with encouragement of them to get it done. Taking frequent breaks while working helps children with ADHD replenish their attention span and self-motivation so they can concentrate better, persist, and complete the next small quota of work you assign to them. (If this feels like an exasperating consumption of time, keep in mind it's a more constructive way to use the time you'd otherwise spend on nagging the child to get the work done. Also keep in mind the suggestion from Principle 4 that, when it comes to situations that often create conflict with your child, you're wise to start with the end in mind. How do you want to end this homework session or other work period? With yelling from you and crying from your child or relative peace and a child who has the satisfaction of a job finished and maybe even well done?)

If you find that your child or teen cannot get through the small quota you have assigned without getting off task, consider making the work quota even smaller. It's all a matter of finding out what your child's attention span for this type of work actually is and breaking down the work so that the quotas you assign fit within it.

2. Break down the task into intervals of time. You can ask a young child with ADHD to work for 3, 4, or 5 minutes, then give her a 1-minute break, then assign another 5 minutes of work. For older children, you can stretch this time interval to 10 minutes of work with a 3-minute break and then another 10 minutes of assigned work. This method can suit some tasks better than others, such as cleaning up a room, emptying the dishwasher, setting the table, or doing work in the yard or garden. All of these chores or tasks involve work that is harder to divide up into equal quotas of work in the way that you can divide up things like math problems, which involve more discrete units of work, and lend themselves better to time-based work periods.

3. Make the check-ins unpredictable. If you're not breaking up the task, as with monitoring your child's work to encourage his own awareness, it helps to time your accountability check-ins somewhat randomly. When your child doesn't know when you're going to check in, her best strategy is to behave well or stay on task and keep working on what she was assigned to do if she wants to maximize the positive attention and rewards from you.

4. Consider using a baby monitor to keep tabs on your child. If you can see and/or hear that your child appears to be losing focus on the task that has been assigned, you know to go into your child's room right away and provide a supervisory checkup. Many parents have told me that showing up the minute the child drifts off task helps to keep their child accountable

5. Accountability checks aren't just for work, and they're not just correcting your child. Even when not doing some sort of work, your child with ADHD will need more frequent supervision and accountability for his actions than other children, whether he's just playing, watching TV, or working on some craft project. Check-ins for all these situations help make children more accountable for their behavior and also reassure you that they are safe and being well behaved, both of which are more problematic for a child with ADHD. Just be sure to offer praise and simple affection as well as encouragement to keep it up when you catch the child behaving well and following the rules. If instead the child is misbehaving, you may have to impose a negative consequence, such as loss of tokens or points or a privilege the child expected later that day. For even worse infractions, a period of time-out might have to be invoked. Wherever possible, reinforce the positive, but holding your child accountable includes imposing consequences for the negative too.

6. Include someone else in your accountability plan. Sharing success with someone we care about can provide us with greater incentives to get our work done or follow through on doing something we agreed to do. So let your child know that, when she has completed the assigned task or behaved well in any situation that you're monitoring, you'll take a picture on your phone, and you and the child together will send the photo to someone your child cares about, such as the other parent, a favorite aunt or uncle, or a grandparent.

Improving Accountability with a Behavior Report Card

There are times when you cannot be around your child to supervise him frequently—when your child is with a babysitter, playing at another child's home, in a religious education class, or attending some organized club, sport, or other event like scouts. You can hold your child more accountable for his actions when he's not with you by using a Behavior Report Card.

You can make copies of the card shown on the facing page (or see the end of the table of contents for information on how to download and print copies) or just make your own on your computer. In the version of the card shown, I've specified a variety of behaviors that children with

Behavior Report Card

Child's Name _____ Date _____

Supervisor _____ Event _____

Instructions: Please rate this child's behavior from 1 (poor) to 5 (excellent) for each period in the columns below. Each period = _____ minutes

Behaviors	Periods					
	1	2	3	4	5	6
Pays Attention to Supervisor						
Obeys Instructions						
Gets Along Well with Other Children						
Controls Emotions Well for Age						
Shows Good Impulse Control for Age						
Gets Along Well with Supervisor						

From *12 Principles for Raising a Child with ADHD* by Russell A. Barkley. Copyright © 2021 The Guilford Press.

ADHD typically have difficulty with in various situations. The remaining columns are numbered and usually represent a specific time period, such as every 15, 20, or 30 minutes. This is how often your child is to be rated by the supervisor during this event or activity. But the time period here doesn't have to be exact. These are rough guidelines for when to evaluate. Essentially, the rating should occur when the supervisor has time in the midst of carrying out his or her other responsibilities. The person supervising that event or situation can briefly rate the child's behavior using a scale from 1 (poor) to 5 (excellent). Younger children need more frequent supervision, feedback, and rating than older children, so specify shorter intervals for them, maybe even going down to 15-minute periods. Of course, the frequency of the evaluation must also be based on the type of event in which your child is participating and how often the adult supervising it can take a moment to evaluate your child on this card.

You can leave this card with the supervisor at any event your child is scheduled to attend. Politely ask the supervisor to rate your child on how well he has behaved during that event. Most supervisors appreciate the fact that you want to know how well your child did when under their supervision and that you've provided them with a means of managing that child during the event as well. But be flexible about the timing of the evaluations as such supervisors usually have many other things they have to accomplish if this is an organized activity of some kind.

When you pick up your child after this event, take a moment right then to briefly review the card with the supervisor (if he or she has time) and your child. What was the supervisor's overall impression? Then speak with your child privately about the various ratings on the card. Focus on the most positive behaviors first. Praise your child for how well he did in that area of conduct. Then focus on the more negative behaviors. Ask your child what happened or went wrong that led to that low rating. Then ask what he could do next time to get a better rating. All of this conversation is intended to increase ownership of behavior, self-evaluation, and being accountable. Then add up the total points on the card. These are reward points that your child can use to buy special privileges from you.

Of course, you must make up a reward menu to go with this card system. (See Principle 7 for instructions.) If you've already set one up, then just use that reward system with the points earned on this report card going toward the purchase of privileges set up in that home point system. Go down the list and determine how much each privilege should cost in terms of points to be earned on the behavior report card.

Also, consider the possibility of using a card like this one yourself with your child during special events, such as when company comes to visit, or another child comes over to play with your child, or you have gone to a party, club, or sporting event with your child, in which case you become the supervisor. You can just make up a card and specify on the card the sorts of behavior you will be monitoring. So, think creatively about how to use this card system. It can be adapted to virtually any situation in which you want to monitor your child's behavior more closely and reward him for how well he behaved.

You can also use this report card to monitor your child's behavior at school and help improve school conduct and performance by linking it to a home reward program, such as a point or token system. Full instructions for doing this can be found in my comprehensive book *Taking Charge of ADHD, Fourth Edition.*

Using the Behavior Report Card for Self-Evaluation

After a few weeks of using the behavior report card in a particular situation, consider shifting to having your child rate herself on the card. You simply have your child or teen fill out the report card periodically during the activity (or in one without supervision). Your child rates herself on the list of target behaviors that are to be the focus of this card system. Within a supervised activity, your child must show the card to the supervising adult to see if the adult concurs with the self-ratings. This review can also offer an opportunity for further discussion between the child and supervisor about how things went during that activity and what could be done better next time. After a few weeks of using the card for self-evaluations, it could be used less frequently or eliminated altogether if behavior in that situation is now no longer a problem.

Improving Accountability through Social Commitments

For older children and especially teens with ADHD (or any teen for that matter), an effective means for increasing the likelihood that they will do something they have promised to do is to commit to doing it with someone else. Think about exercising as a good example. You could agree to start running on your own to improve your health. But studies show you are far more likely to actually engage in this exercise regularly if you commit to doing it with another person. Friends, neighbors, coworkers, relatives, and even members you meet at your health club can all serve this role for you. I recall when I first began running as a form of exercise when I was in my 20s. I found I was much more likely to get out of bed early before work and go for a run if I did so with my like-minded next-door neighbor. I also trained for longer runs, and even several marathons, on the weekends, with a close friend and coworker.

Your older child or teen is no different. How he is perceived and valued by others in his life can be a highly motivating source for engaging in self-improvement programs and completing work commitments. So, think about your child or teen's friends, classmates, or other neighborhood children. Could they somehow serve as a means to help improve your child's likelihood of doing, and accountability for doing certain things? Could your child study or do homework several times each week with a friend from the same class who has the same homework or class project to do? Could your teen study for an important exam with a friend or classmate who has to study for the same exam? In any of these scenarios where you may be having another child or teen on hand for your child to work with, be sure that this is a teen of good character who will inspire your child to work more productively and not someone whose behavior can also be problematic. That could prove disastrous as the children merely serve as distractions for each other and no work actually gets done. Maybe you would be well off hiring a tutor to work with your child several afternoons each week on a subject in which she is struggling at school. Again, your child is more likely to study, work hard, and improve if she is accountable to another person—in this case, her tutor.

If your child or teen wants to join an organized sport or club, is there someone the child knows who could join with him and thus be more likely to participate in that organized activity? A parent can also serve in this role. But research shows that children and teens value the impressions of peers much more than those of their parents. And that is why their peers are so much more likely to motivate them to complete projects or engage in self-improvement than a parent or sibling would be.

Improving Accountability by Clarifying Household Rules and Enforcing Them Consistently

Sometimes we contribute to our children's difficulties being responsible and held accountable for their actions because the rules we expect them to follow are not always clear. More likely, we have stipulated the rules of our house but don't enforce them consistently. We may even break them ourselves, all the while telling our children to still obey the rule (do as we say, not as we do).

To improve the clarity of our household rules, it can help immensely to write down the most common ones on a chart, especially those most frequently broken by the child or teen with ADHD. Make a poster of the rules in the house that seem to be violated most often and post this on the front of the refrigerator or some other highly visible location. Now there are no excuses for not knowing the rules.

Yet the real trick here is to enforce them consistently. There can be no accountability or responsibility when rules are applied sporadically or with favoritism, or can be avoided or escaped through arguing with a parent or blaming someone else for the rule violation. So, this poster is as much a cue to parents that these rules are to be enforced religiously (consistently) within the family as it is a reminder to the children in the household. It's also a reminder to parents to provide appropriate consequences for following or violating the rules. Some parents find it helpful to specify on the chart how many points or tokens a child can earn or lose toward privileges for obeying and disobeying these rules.

Another way to improve the clarity and consistency of rules in the household is through the Transition Plan discussed in Principle 12. Setting up and reviewing the rules of a situation or activity with your child or teen just before starting into that activity clearly helps improve accountability and compliance. And explaining the rewards that a child can earn in that situation and the negative consequences that will occur if they break the rules is a further means of improving accountability by making it crystal clear what is going to happen in that situation if rules are or are not followed. Providing frequent feedback throughout the activity is another way to strengthen accountability in a child or teen with ADHD.

I started this chapter talking about your child's executive functions and how they make Principle 6 so valuable to parents of children with ADHD. I'd also like to end with executive functions. When we talk about the need to be aware of our own behavior and reflect on how that behavior is or is not serving our goals, we're really describing metacognition. In some schemes, metacognition is the most sophisticated executive function of all and one that develops over years, possibly maturing fully only once children are into their 20s. With this understanding, you wouldn't expect any 7-year-old to have the insight to see exactly where she has gone wrong and how she could change that in the future. Metacognition develops with a lot of coaching and experience, and for children with ADHD the process may take even longer and require even more assistance from parents, teachers, and other adults. Therefore it makes sense to get started now, but it also makes sense not to expect too much from a young child—or even a teenager—with ADHD.

TOUCH MORE, REWARD MORE, AND TALK LESS

Ask any parent, "What's the biggest challenge in raising a child with ADHD?" and you're likely to hear some variation on "Getting my child to do what he's supposed to do." The fact that children with ADHD have such a hard time starting, sticking to, and completing tasks often leads parents to spend much of their day issuing commands, requests, and reminders. As noted in Principle 4, this is a recipe for conflict and a good reason for prioritizing what really needs to get done so you can cut down on the number of orders you deliver to your child.

Cultivating your child's self-awareness and teaching your child to become accountable (eventually), à la Principle 6, can help your child do what he's supposed to do, but you still have to scaffold the entire process, being aware of what's going on with your child in a mindful way (Principle 5) and also learning the best way to verbally direct your child when you really do have to tell her to get to work and get it done. In this chapter I'll show you how to make those requests and also how to add some incentives so that your child won't need the nagging that sometimes feels unavoidable.

> **THE PROBLEM:** Parents of children with ADHD talk too much.

If you've read Principle 6, you know that I'm all for some types of parental talk. The social narration, evaluations of your own behavior out loud, and casual conversations that have been not-so-casually engineered to nudge your child toward self-awareness are important strategies for parents of children with ADHD. Where many parents of kids with ADHD go overboard, however, is in the constant stream of commands, harangues, and pleas to do something. You likely recognize that you talk way too much to your child or teen with ADHD. You know it's not working if your child isn't listening to or obeying what you say. But maybe you keep at it just because you don't know what else to do. Principle 4 gave you one thing to do—reconsider your priorities and let go of some of the small stuff you ask your child to do. But what about those times when your child really does have to get something done and all your words get you nowhere?

Does this scenario sound familiar? You're having company in about an hour, and you've just discovered that your recently cleaned and neatened living room has been trashed by your child with ADHD. So, despite your exasperation, you ask him nicely to put away his toys, and he says, "OK, Mom, just a minute." You come back in a few minutes to find your child still playing in the middle of the mess, so you repeat your request, this time saying that company's coming in just a few minutes and your son needs to start cleaning up right now. He says "OK, OK," and you leave— only to find nothing changed when you return a few minutes later. This time you explain that Aunt Minnie and Uncle Manny are old and will trip on those little action figures and hurt themselves and he really needs to put them away. No luck. So next you add a threat, maybe that now little Morty won't be allowed to play video games in his room while the adults chat if he doesn't get moving this instant. When that fails, you repeat all this again but with a raised, sterner voice. Perhaps you now try to get your partner to enter the fray in hopes that he can be more convincing at getting this chore done or that two of you are more convincing than one.

Throughout all this your child is essentially ignoring you, eventually fighting back with indignation of his own and pleas in response to your pleas. As your voice and emotions intensify, so do your child's. Now your explanation has become a full-fledged argument—one you won't win. And still you keep talking. It's as if parents trying to get compliance from a child with ADHD think he has information deficit disorder and that more and more words will correct the problem.

But they won't. In the Introduction you learned why children with ADHD aren't going to be able to more effectively control their own behavior just because you've provided extensive explanations of why they need to do what you're asking:

■ Language doesn't work well at controlling their behavior. The part of the brain where language interacts with and guides behavior is just not functioning as well as it does in other children.

■ They have a disorder of performance (doing what they know) rather than one of knowledge (knowing what to do). So, no amount of information is going to work well at getting them to listen and obey.

■ They have a self-motivation deficit. That means that when they must activate and sustain their behavior to do something that is not fun or rewarding to do, they are less likely to either start it or complete it. Stick-to-itiveness is just not their forte.

■ They are highly distractible, especially when doing work. Anything around them that may be more interesting or entertaining to do than the work you've assigned to them is likely to capture their attention and behavior, causing them to get off task yet again.

■ Their deficit in working memory (remembering what they are supposed to be doing) can make it hard to complete the task you requested.

■ About 65% of children with ADHD also have oppositional defiant disorder. They develop behaviors involving stubbornness, ignoring, talking back to you, arguing, verbally defying you, even physically resisting your efforts to get them to do as you ask.

What is a parent to do when faced with all this?

THE SOLUTION: Touch more, talk less.

Whenever you must ask your child to do something for you, or praise her for what she's done, or reprimand her for something she has not done or has done wrong, try doing the following:

1. Go to the child. Don't try talking to him from far away—up a flight of stairs, across a room, or from another room on the same floor. The farther away you are, the less effective your words and actions are likely to be. So go stand next to your child before speaking to him.

2. Touch the child. Put your hand on your child's shoulder, arm, or hand, or touch the child's chin gently with your finger. Whatever gesture you feel comfortable using will convey your affection for your child and get her attention. Children differ in what touches they will perceive as signs of intimacy and love and what they will perceive as unpleasant, so of course use your knowledge of your child here. But whatever you do, touch the child, as this will greatly personalize your interaction while showing your affection.

3. Look into your child's eyes. Whenever possible, look directly at your child rather than talking to the back or top of his head. Most people find that eye contact increases the impact and importance of an interaction, and children are no different. Yes, some children are shy, socially anxious, or on the autism spectrum, any of which makes it harder for them to make eye contact with others. Or it might cause them to briefly look away from you, finding your direct gaze unnerving. But at least initially make eye contact with the child to make a connection mind to mind.

4. Briefly say what needs to be said. Use short, direct phrases! No more and no less. Keep what you have to say brief and to the point. If you want something done, say it precisely and firmly: "I want you to pick up your toys now." (To avoid getting into a whole new series of repeated requests and wrangling over whether the job you've assigned actually has been done as you instructed, see the box on the next page.)

- *If giving a direction or command,* be sure to use a businesslike tone of voice that clearly conveys that you mean what you say. Don't yell; just be direct and firm.

- *If you came to thank or praise your child,* make it pleasant, sincere, and brief, and make it count: "I really like it when you listen to me and do as I ask" or "Thank you for helping me unload the dishwasher and put the dishes away." But mean it. Be genuine, approving, and affectionate in tone, without exaggeration. Children, like adults, are quick to spot insincere praise.

- *If it is a reprimand,* sound firm or even stern but keep your voice low yet forceful. Don't scream or yell or convey anger—be direct and disapproving but not out of control. Again, keep it short and to the point, no matter what it is you are trying to say. Talk less, touch more, and do it one on one.

Head Off Arguments with Chore Cards

If your child is old enough to have jobs to do around the home and can read, you may find it useful to make up a chore card for each job. Using a 3″ × 5″ file card or something similar, list the steps involved in correctly doing that chore. Then, when you want your child to do the chore, simply hand the child the card and state that this is what you want done. These cards can greatly reduce the amount of arguing that occurs about whether a child has done a job or chore properly. You might also indicate on the card how much time it should take to get it done and then set your kitchen timer for this length of time so the child knows exactly when it is to be finished.

5. Have your child repeat an instruction or directive back to you. Ask your child to tell you what you have just asked her to do. A child is more likely to comply with a command or instruction repeated back to you. So simply say, "What did I just ask you to do?" in a kind voice.

6. Depart with affection. Before taking your hand off your child and departing, give him a gentle squeeze, soft rub, light pat, or kiss on the head . You want to convey concern, affection, and intimacy in a personal way even if you expressed disapproval for something the child failed to do or did wrong. Especially then, what you wish to signal is that your disapproval is a response to what he did, not who he is. Your child needs to know that you don't dislike him, just the unacceptable behavior.

Research shows that communicating in this way is much more effective with children who have ADHD than the reflexive ways we typically give instructions to our children. But children with ADHD also often need more salient and immediate consequences, such as rewards, in addition to verbal praise or correction/disapproval.

> **THE PROBLEM:** Internal self-motivation is weak.

Children and teens with ADHD struggle mightily to sustain their attention and work-related behavior toward assigned tasks. While this can be due to being distractible, a big factor is their deficit in internal motivation. We all need self-motivation, one of the executive functions described in the Introduction, when (1) we're faced with work that we don't find interesting, enjoyable, rewarding, or otherwise engaging and (2) there is no immediate consequence for getting the work done. It's important to compensate for this deficit in self-motivation because your child with ADHD, like all children, will encounter more and more scut work as he gets older. Right now he might have trouble sticking with unrewarding activities like schoolwork, chores, and personal hygiene, and if he can't learn to motivate himself to get these things done, he'll have even more trouble with a job, personal finances, property maintenance, and even raising his own children.

Research dating back to the 1970s has shown that children and teens with ADHD can't persist at activities that don't provide some degree of immediate reward, entertainment, or intrinsic interest to them. There are two problems here:

1. The usual rewards and motivations that we often associate with schoolwork and chores are too weak for children with ADHD. Scientists have shown that the brain networks and neurochemicals associated with reward are smaller, less sensitive, and more erratic or variable in those with ADHD. So such things as grades and certificates for school work, desiring to be a good student and gain peer and teacher recognition for doing so, the admiration of others, contributing to our family and society, and learning to be a responsible and self-motivated employee in our first jobs are typically not strong enough to motivate the child with ADHD.

This is not to say your child does not find some work intrinsically interesting. We all vary in the sorts of tasks and activities we enjoy, and children with ADHD are no different. We've found that many of the activities that children and teens with ADHD often enjoy involve movement, such as in sports, physical or manual activities, creative expression like performing arts, and engaging with others directly, often competitively, or through social media. But those with ADHD are as diverse as the rest of the population, and some may find arcane subjects interesting, such as weather, animals or insects, technology, or specific topics in history. If they find a task or activity interesting in some way, they'll more easily start and stick with that activity.

2. Consequences have to be immediate and frequent to sustain their behavior toward a task. In Principle 8 we'll get into the problems that children with ADHD have with time, but for now what's important to know is that long delays before consequences are delivered are a serious problem in ADHD. The longer the delay, the less valuable the consequence will be to your child. And while this is true of typical children as well, the degree to which those with ADHD discount or devalue the delayed consequences are markedly greater. If you want to see a child with ADHD fail to get something done, just assign some boring work for which there is no immediate payoff. You will be fighting with the child to keep her on task until the work gets done, if it ever does. No wonder children and teens with ADHD find video games, particularly Internet-based competitive gaming, to be so addictive. Indeed, 15–20% of teens with ADHD qualify as having an Internet or gaming addiction. These games have everything that a term paper or weekend chore lacks: intrinsic appeal and constant immediate rewards.

> **THE SOLUTION:** Use frequent, immediate, external rewards.

So just as there were two problems related to motivation, so there are two solutions.

Use Powerful Artificial Rewards

By powerful I mean highly motivating. And by artificial, I mean rewards that are not ordinarily associated with doing that task. As much as you may not like to do so, it's essential that you employ lots of artificial external rewards to activate your child with ADHD to work and then motivate her to sustain that work long enough to get it done. Many parents worry that doing this will amount to bribing their child to do what others do without reward and that the child will never learn to do the task for its own sake or for some larger social reward, like admiration, status, and approval. The problem is the child with ADHD is simply not going to *be* motivated by intrinsic rewards, so you're not really at risk here of replacing some desirable internal motivation with some materialistic, artificial external one. Think of these external rewards as the equivalent for children with ADHD of ramps, hearing aids, mechanical limbs, canes and walkers, and glasses for the physically, hearing, or sight impaired—a necessary prosthesis to overcome a disability so it is not so impairing.

As Stephen Covey said in his *7 Habits of Highly Effective People,* "Think win/win." Getting the work done is a win for you, but it's rarely a win for your child, so make it one: When any sort of work has to be done, think about what you can offer to motivate your child to get it done. What does your child like to do, or have, or consume? Can you easily make it available when the child accomplishes the assigned work?

You can also think about this strategy as an employment contract. Like your employer, who offers you a fair day's pay for a fair day's work, you're offering your child a small reward for getting a chore or homework assignment done. In the process, you're teaching your child a valuable lesson that she can take into her own future employment: everyone's time and effort are valuable.

One of the easiest ways to have rewards readily available when you need them is to create a home token program or point system. These systems, described in full in the fourth edition of my book *Taking Charge of ADHD,* allows your child to earn tokens for work done and then cash them in, like money, to purchase privileges. The box on pages 110–111 offers a concise summary of how a token or point program works.

Make Feedback and Rewards Immediate and Frequent

If the second problem that children and teens with ADHD have is with the delay before a consequence or reward is given, then the solution is quite simply to reduce or eliminate the delay. The child or teen with ADHD needs to know often during task performance exactly how she's doing. And she needs to obtain her rewards much more frequently throughout the task than a typical child or teen.

I find it helpful to think of our self-motivation as similar to a car's fuel tank. The car can have the best GPS and equipment to get it to its destination, but it's not going anywhere without fuel. Likewise, a person can have the best plans and best tools for completing those plans, but nothing is getting done without self-motivation—our willpower is that fuel. You can see this in the figure on the next page, which shows the executive function fuel tank on the left, and on the right things that research has shown are likely to replenish and sustain our self-motivation while working—our self-regulation and persistence. The list that follows describes the methods for replenishing the EF fuel tank.

Replenishing the Executive Function Fuel Tank

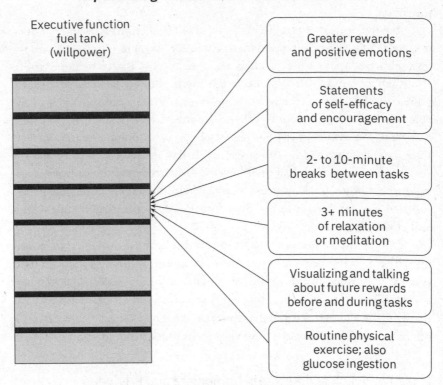

Executive function
fuel tank
(willpower)

Greater rewards
and positive emotions

Statements
of self-efficacy
and encouragement

2- to 10-minute
breaks between tasks

3+ minutes
of relaxation
or meditation

Visualizing and talking
about future rewards
before and during tasks

Routine physical
exercise; also
glucose ingestion

The suggestions for replenishing executive function are adapted from the research summarized in I. M. Bauer and R. F. Baumeister (2011). Self-Regulatory Strength. In K. Vohs and R. F. Baumeister (Eds.), *Handbook of Self-Regulation* (2nd ed., pp. 64–82). New York: Guilford Press.

Ways to Replenish the EF Fuel Tank and Motivate Your Child to Work

Use rewards often. Your child will run out of fuel faster than kids who don't have ADHD, so keep those rewards coming to keep the child on track. One of the best ways to provide frequent rewards with less likelihood the child may get bored with any specific one is to use a token or point system, as explained in the box on pages 110–111.

Use self-talk. Self-speech can be a useful tool to assist us in motivating ourselves to do otherwise uninteresting work. Have your child with ADHD talk out loud softly to himself about the goal while working and what he will earn when done. He can also give himself positive encouragement—a pep talk. We call these statements of self-efficacy—essentially, "I CAN do this!" Like a football coach before a big game, you can encourage your child to tell himself that he can do this, that he has the talent and the skills, and that nothing can stop him from winning the reward.

Break down the work. You met this idea in Principle 6. Cutting the work down into smaller units and then taking frequent breaks of 2–10 minutes depending on how long the work period is helps all of us to refuel our tanks and stay motivated to finish the task. At your job, you might do 20 minutes of work that requires concentration, get up and get a coffee, do another 20 minutes of work, get up and stretch or walk around, and so forth. Each short break allows you to rest your EF brain, move about, get a brief reward, then return to work with more motivation to work than when you started on your short break. Your child is no different. Frequent breaks help restore motivational fuel to get work done.

Take a mindfulness pause before working. Before starting a new task, it can help to take a 3-minute break and just relax for a moment or even use mindfulness meditation to power down our current EF brain and its thoughts and emotions. (See Principle 5.) Doing so allows us to prepare our minds for what we may want to do next. See the Resources to find books that can teach you how to coach your child in using mindfulness to help her calm down, clear her mind of negative thoughts, and just prepare her mind to deal with what she will be doing next.

Visualize reaching the goal and enjoying the reward. Just before she starts the assigned work, have your child visualize completing the task and receiving the reward you've promised. Suggest that she try to think of how good it will feel to have the work done and to be enjoying the reward.

Use a picture of the reward. Better yet, if your child is working for some sort of tangible reward, like a toy or snack item, or a privilege that can be easily pictured, look for a picture of this on the Internet, print it out, and place it in front of the child to help motivate him to stay on task and complete the job.

Exercise often. Studies also show that both children and adults can improve their powers of concentration, persistence, and willpower by

Setting Up the Home Poker Chip Program or Point System

THE HOME POKER CHIP PROGRAM (FOR AGES 4–8)

1. Get a set of plastic poker chips and assign a value to the chips (1 point for each chip of any color for ages 4–5, different values for different colors for ages 6–8).

2. Explain to your child that you feel he has not been rewarded enough for doing nice things at home and you want to set up a new reward program so he can earn privileges and things for behaving properly.

3. Make a "nice bank" together for the chips earned. Have some fun decorating it with your child.

4. Together, make up a list of the 10–15 privileges you want your child to earn with the poker chips—both occasional special privileges like going to a movie or out to a restaurant or game parlor and the everyday privileges your child takes for granted (TV, video games, etc.).

5. Make up a second list of jobs and chores you often ask your child to perform—household chores such as setting the table, self-care tasks like brushing teeth before bed, and any other self-help tasks you give the child that normally pose a problem for you.

6. Decide how many chips each job or chore is worth. For 4- and 5-year-olds, assign from one to three chips for most tasks, and perhaps five for really big jobs. For 6- to 8-year-olds, use a range of 1 to 10 chips, and perhaps give a larger amount for big jobs. Remember, the harder the job, the more chips you will pay.

7. Take a moment and add up approximately how many chips you think your child will earn in a typical day if she does most of these jobs. Then decide how many chips your child should have to pay for each of the rewards you listed. Usually two-thirds of the child's daily chips should be spent on typical daily privileges. This allows the child to save about one-third of her chips every day toward the purchase of some of the very special rewards on the list.

8. Tell your child that he will have a chance to earn "bonus" chips when he performs a chore in a nice, prompt, and pleasant manner. Give these when your child has done a job in an especially pleasant and prompt manner.

9. Tell the child that chips will be given only for jobs that are done on the first request. If you have to repeat a command to the child, she will not receive any chips for doing it.

10. Finally, be sure to go out of your way this week to give chips away for any small appropriate behavior. Remember, you can reward a child even for good behaviors that are not on the list of jobs. Be alert for opportunities to reward the child.

Note: Do not take chips away this week for misbehavior!!!

THE HOME POINT SYSTEM (FOR AGES 8 AND OVER)

1. Get a notebook and set it up like a checkbook with five columns, one each for the date, the item, deposits, withdrawals, and the running balance. When your child is rewarded with points, write the job in under "item" and enter the amount as a "deposit." Add it to the child's balance. When your child buys a privilege with his points, note the privilege under "item," place this amount in the "withdrawal" column, and deduct this amount from the "balance." The program works just like the chip system except that points are recorded in the book instead of using poker chips.

2. Follow the chip program, but use a range of 5–25 points for most daily jobs and up to 200 points for very big jobs. Typically, you might consider paying 15 points for every 15 minutes of extended work a child has to do. Only parents are to write in the point notebook.

engaging in routine physical exercise. So if your child is not yet involved in any sort of routinely scheduled sports or exercise programs, consider starting one. It doesn't have to be an organized sport; just daily walking or running can facilitate our capacity to attend to and persist at work.

Consume small sips of sugared beverages. Finally, there is some evidence, at least with adults, that consuming small amounts of sugar-containing fluids periodically during a mentally demanding task can help us sustain our effort. The brain runs on blood glucose (a sugar), so keeping our blood sugar level somewhat elevated can facilitate brain functioning, particularly when it comes to self-control. So think about allowing your child to sip on some lemonade or a sports drink periodically while working. I said *sip*. This does not mean quaffing mass quantities of these beverages as that clearly has a downside, contributing as it can to obesity and poor dental hygiene, as well as sleepiness. If your child can't handle a glass or bottle of the drink without drinking it all at once, use plastic cups with lids that have straws or a sports water bottle with the protruding nipple that limits how much can be consumed in one sip. You can also simply give smaller amounts of the beverage each time and replenish that small amount while your child is working.

Can Providing External Rewards Teach Your Child to Self-Motivate?

As you know, most adults need to get paid to go to work every day and do their job as expected. We don't necessarily outgrow the need for external rewards. But does that mean that children with ADHD will never learn to motivate themselves? Of course not. The hope is that as they get older, they will internalize the methods you've used to motivate them and come up with their own. Teenagers often get very good at the self-talk that sticking with a task like a term paper requires. Or they come up with their own small rewards they can earn after each chunk of work (like a couple of their favorite chips after every paragraph written for the term paper or 5 minutes on their favorite video game in between pages).

This is not to say that your child with ADHD will never need those extrinsic rewards to get through onerous or boring tasks. (Who among us adults does not need them?) With your loving support and persistent coaching, you'll pass on the motivational strategies, and they will mature with your child. (My book *Taking Charge of Adult ADHD* offers ideas for translating many of the strategies I use with children for the grown-up world.) But I can't stress how important it is to apply this entire idea appropriately. Watch out not to overdo the rewards in these ways:

1. Don't offer your child rewards for *everything*. Some things you want your child to do will be motivating enough that you don't have to offer up some kind of material reward or privilege for doing it. Letting your child help you while you're baking, grocery shopping (pushing the cart, selecting specific items from shelves, etc.), gardening, or doing other chores can sometimes be fun for your child in its own right. There may also be types of schoolwork or other chores at home that your child *does* find intrinsically interesting, such as working on a certain topic in science or history or even certain features of math. Every child is different, so what every child finds intrinsically interesting enough to sustain his curiosity and work will be different.

There is some research evidence, though not consistent, to suggest that when you reward typical children for things they already find interesting to do, such as reading certain books for pleasure, you may cause a decline in their motivation to purse these activities once you withdraw those external rewards. Perhaps it's because the child came to focus on the more obvious and powerful external motivators you were providing that replaced the lesser intrinsic ones. Or perhaps paying the child to do something she likes cheapens the task for her in some way. Whatever the explanation, it's possible to provide so much of a reward, and so frequently, that it comes to interfere with learning better work habits and acquiring intrinsic motivation to do things. It is far less clear if this applies to children with ADHD who already suffer from deficits in internal motivation. But it's still a good point to keep in mind even when assisting your own child with ADHD: don't reward her so much for things she already finds enjoyable to do on her own; save the artificial rewards for the tasks she struggles to complete.

It might be easy to get carried away with the token or points system (see the box on pages 110–111) once it starts to work—you may be tempted to put every single thing that you ask of your child on the list. We used to joke that in certain families the child had to earn tokens for doing virtually everything except breathing—and even that was up for consideration! Seriously, though, some parents wanted to require their child to earn rewards for nearly every behavior required of the child, earning virtually every privilege available to the child in the household. The result was that the child was nearly suffocating psychologically from the intensity of the program and the demand that he had to earn everything he wanted to do. The result in such rare cases was that the child lost all interest in the reward program or stressed out over all the things he had to earn through the token system.

Instead, cut your child a little slack and let her have some privileges, physical rewards like snacks or small toys, for just existing and being part of the family. Affection, approval, respect, dignity, and unconditional positive regard are part of natural family relationships. Giving our children special favors and activities should be noncontingent at times, meaning that the child should not have to do anything to be blessed with them. Stick to using the reward system to motivate your child to do the things that have not been getting done and really need to be done.

2. Make sure your child doesn't become obsessed with earning the rewards. Is your child starting to hoard tokens or points, refusing to use them for privileges? I've seen this on enough occasions to at least forewarn parents of the possibility. If it happens to you, set up a "use it or lose it" policy such that the child has to spend a certain amount of her income from her tokens or points each week or it will be taken from her bank account anyway.

3. Be careful that the rewards don't start to distract your child from the task. I've found this to be most common with younger children with ADHD, such as those in kindergarten or first grade. We set up a token system in the kindergarten classes I had designed and managed as part of a clinical research study. Children with ADHD could earn poker chips for the various types of work we were asking them to do. They could also earn them for following class rules, doing as instructed, and interacting well with other children. It all seemed so reasonable in theory. Yet in practice we found that placing poker chips on the desks of the children who earned the reward subsequently distracted them from doing additional work or paying attention to what the teacher was teaching. Instead, the children started playing with the chips, counting them, stacking them, talking about what they would spend them on during the next "reward exchange break," when they could cash them in for various classroom privileges. Other researchers in the field at that time had also noted this problem.

One solution we came up with was to pin small pouches made of plain-colored fabric to the backs of the children's shirts or sweaters. Then when the teacher gave them a token for following instructions, working, or other good behavior, she showed it to them, placed it in their back pouch, and gave them an affectionate squeeze or pat on the shoulder. This kept the tokens out of sight and prevented them from becoming the sole focus of the child's train of thought at the moment.

MAKE TIME REAL

As explained briefly in the Introduction, children with ADHD seem to be blind to time. More specifically, they are nearsighted toward the future. They have a huge problem with sensing and using time, which makes it very difficult for them to manage their time. This is one of the most important discoveries made about the nature of ADHD over the past few decades, and it has enormous ramifications for your child.

> **THE PROBLEM:** Time escapes children with ADHD.

As you've undoubtedly noticed, children with ADHD seem to be unable to see and deal with anything that isn't currently happening around them—the now. All children develop a sense of time, but it doesn't happen all at once. And because it happens mentally with few visible signs of its development initially, it can be hard to tell if anything is going wrong with it. But something is going wrong, as will become evident when tasks involving time and timeliness start to get assigned to your child.

How Children Develop a Sense of Time

The older children become, the further ahead in time they can anticipate likely events and prepare for them. The youngest children can anticipate what's likely to happen only a few minutes ahead. By elementary school, this foresight may extend to a few hours, and by middle childhood it may be 8–12 hours. It then advances to a few days in adolescence and a few weeks in late adolescence and early adulthood. By age 30 or so, the average time period over which adults make typical decisions about preparing for their future is 8–12 weeks.

First comes hindsight. A sense of time seems to start with the child's being able to look backward. Faced with an unfamiliar situation, most children stop and think about events they've experienced that may be relevant to what's happening right now before they decide how to act.

Then comes foresight. As they mature and they accumulate more and more knowledge about past sequences of events, they start to use this store of knowledge to anticipate what may happen next. This is the beginning of foresight. Over development, their capacity for foresight grows and their window on time, or time horizon, pushes further out into the future. This lets them think about, anticipate, and, most importantly, act to prepare for future events.

What's Going On with Children Who Have ADHD?

Children with ADHD don't seem to use this combination of hindsight and foresight very well. They're less likely to even stop to think about their past because they're very impulsive. And without the benefit of the past experiences that might have informed them about how to behave right now, they don't learn the importance of using foresight to anticipate the future. Instead they make snap decisions based largely on their feelings in the moment.

As the parent of a child with ADHD, you know how well that works out. Your child seems to ricochet around like a pinball, reacting to one immediate event after another without ever seeing what might be ahead or whether he could do something to guide his own course rather than be at the mercy of fleeting impulses. Unfortunately, those who don't understand the time blindness that is part of ADHD often believe the child just doesn't care about the consequences of his actions. They may view this behavior as a conscious choice flowing from some moral failing rather than as a neurological problem that leaves the child lacking the ability to even consider the future.

Children with ADHD can't look as far ahead as others. It's an exaggeration, fortunately, to say that children with ADHD can't think about or deal with anything but the now. As they grow up, they develop the ability to think about and anticipate the future, but just not as far ahead as other children of the same age (see the figure comparing typical children with ADHD children in the Introduction). This problem with perceiving, thinking about, and dealing with time and the future continues into adulthood—people with ADHD are routinely less able to deal with the time, timing, and timeliness of events and their actions in daily life. Of course, this also means they will be much less likely to engage in time management, which is essentially how we manage ourselves relative to time, deadlines, promises about the future, and likely future events.

This is a major and serious problem, because as children grow up, they are expected to deal effectively with time-dependent responsibilities like deadlines, promises, commitments, goals, assignments, and appointments. Indeed, the older children become, the more tasks that involve some element of time and the future they're expected to complete. As a parent you have a close-up view of the problem. In a national survey of children in the United States, I asked parents to rate their children on their executive functions. They reported that their children with ADHD had twice as much trouble with time management as typical children. Most of the children with ADHD were far worse at time management than 93% of typical children! Our studies of adults with ADHD also showed that more than 90% place in the bottom 7% of the population in their ability to engage effectively in time management.

Children with ADHD can't use their sense of time to control their behavior. Apparently the problem is not that these kids have a problem with their *perception* of time. In one study we asked those with ADHD to watch an unlit light bulb. We then turned it on for a short interval and then off again. When we asked them to turn the light on for the same duration, they were usually twice as bad at this task as typical people of the same age. Interestingly, though, the same people with ADHD were able to tell us the length of a sample duration they were shown. It's just that they couldn't use that knowledge to regulate their own behavior in this case, to hold that interval in mind and then reproduce the interval accurately. In short, it is their use of that sense of time in guiding their own behavior while performing a task that is their major problem. Of course, being able to perceive a length of time accurately isn't enough to help you decide what to do if you can't use that sense of time to control yourself.

Time seems to move more slowly in the minds of children with ADHD. It's counterintuitive, but people with ADHD seem to psychologically feel time moving much more slowly than it really is or than other people perceive it as passing. This leads to a couple of significant problems:

▓ *They overestimate the time they have to get something done.* Children with ADHD typically think they have plenty of time to do things they are supposed to do when in reality they have nowhere near as much time as they think. Deadlines, therefore, arrive well ahead of the child's expectations. When your child with ADHD suddenly informs you at bedtime that he needs to create a model of a volcano to take to school the next day, you've undoubtedly reacted with exasperation. You probably couldn't believe your child failed to anticipate this deadline—again. But it's a common manifestation of the time blindness of ADHD: Your child thinks she has more time than she really has to complete an assignment, so she goofs off, gets distracted by other things, or generally wastes some time because she thinks it's OK to do so—she has plenty of time. And then—wham! The actual time period is over, the future has arrived, and your child is nowhere near ready for it.

▓ *They get very impatient when asked to wait.* Children with ADHD are notorious for complaining about having to wait for something to happen and for trying to take shortcuts or get out of the situation that involves waiting. Ask them to line up against a wall in their classroom to get ready to go to lunch. Expect them to fidget, annoy others, elbow their way to the front of the line, or just head straight there. Expect them to horse around, try to pull open the door, whine about the waiting, demand to know how soon they can get going, and otherwise express their impatience with this demand to just wait. Got a long car trip to take with them? Expect them to be insufferable. The common question "Are we there yet?" will be asked incessantly. Having to wait increases not only their impatience and frustration but also their hyperactivity. Fidgeting, squirming, playing with things, touching others, and various antics are likely to increase when they have to wait—it's their way of marking time. And it can be very disruptive, especially in places like school, church, or stores, where they are expected to remain still and there is nothing to do while they are waiting. As one teen with ADHD told me, "Waiting is hell!"

Children with ADHD can't plan when the time horizon for a project is long. Let's take a book report assignment as an example. The instructions might go something like this: "You have 2 weeks to read this book and then turn in a report about it. It will take the teacher a few days to grade the papers, and then you will learn your grade for this assignment." Even typical children struggle with this level of time management and self-organization. But the child with ADHD cannot even manage an interval of 18 seconds very well, and yet he has just been given intervals of 2 days to 2 weeks to manage. Whenever you insert a time delay into any project you ask your child with ADHD to do, you have effectively handicapped him in getting it done. He just won't be able to keep those time intervals in mind and use them to plan ahead and then complete the tasks on his plan when scheduled. As noted in Principle 7, this is one powerful reason that video games have such great appeal to those with ADHD: the time intervals between action and consequence (especially rewards) are very short.

THE SOLUTION: Externalize time, then break it down.

There are a number of very concrete ways to compensate for your child's lack of an internal clock. But before we get to those, here's an important guideline to keep in mind: **Remember that whenever you put a time limit on anything for your child with ADHD you are disabling the child.** That may sound harsh, but it's key to approaching time management with any child who has ADHD. First, let's make one thing very clear: We don't manage time. Time is time. It is a dimension of our physical universe. So when we say that we engage in time management, that is not quite correct. Instead, what we really do (and mean by the term) is we manage our own behavior relative to the flow of time. We try to line up and engage in our actions at the most appropriate times so we can be as effective as possible in carrying out our plans, achieving our goals, and preparing for our future. But, as we've already established, children with ADHD are weak in this capacity. This means that anytime you give your child a time limit to do something, you are automatically disabling her. You are asking her to do something her disorder guarantees she cannot do as well as others her age.

Use External Clocks for Short Tasks

Because their internal clock cannot guide them well when they are doing a task, children with ADHD need to rely more than others on external clocks that show the passage of time, and they need their parents to help them do this. So when you have to ask your child to do a task that involves a relatively short period of time, such as 1 hour or less, you need to put some type of timekeeper in front of him:

A spring-loaded cooking timer. This is the kind Grandma used in the kitchen. You simply give the instruction that involves the time interval ("You have 15 minutes to do _____."), set the timer for that period, and put it in front of the child.

Your own timing device, such as a recording on a digital recorder that counts backward from a specific time interval like 15 or 20 minutes down to zero. Just play it when the child has a task of that length to do. It takes a little time to make it, but its novelty can help children pay attention to the passing of time. That said, a visual representation of time is better than an auditory one.

A smartphone stopwatch timer. Make sure the screen stays visible and doesn't power off after a short interval to save power. I don't like analog (round) alarm clocks as well as digital ones for this particular purpose as they don't show small time intervals very well or how much time has expired and how much is left at a glance. But for longer intervals like 30 minutes to an hour, large analog clocks are fine (see below).

A large Time Timer. This device was designed specifically for people with ADHD. (See the Resources at the end of the book for ordering information.) This is a clock containing a red disk. You can set the timer for up to 1 hour (the clock is now all red), and then as time passes the portion of the disk that is red gets smaller. This is great for doing tasks, chores, homework, or other activities where having a highly visible timekeeper comes in handy. It can also show at a glance just how much time has expired and how much you have left before the deadline.

Downloadable online stopwatches and timer apps for a tablet, iPad, or smartphone. They include traditional clock faces, time bombs, cartoon characters running races, virtual hourglasses, and more. (See the Resources for ordering information.) The trick here is to make sure the timing device is visible while the child is working.

Reduce or Eliminate Time Gaps (Delays) in Assignments for Longer-Term Projects

Whenever there are large gaps in time between instructions, the point where someone needs to comply with them, and then the consequences for persistent compliance, children with ADHD tend to fall apart in their work. (Remember the book report example I gave above?) They don't appreciate how much time they have (or how little), get bored, go "off task," get restless and fidgety, and just become noncompliant. The task never gets completed, and even if completed may never be turned in on time. The solution is another of the ones I suggested in Principle 7: reduce the delays by breaking up the task into smaller chunks, each with its own short time interval (visible) and a reward for completion.

Divide the project up by the number of days until the deadline. Let's take that book report to be done over the next 2 weeks. Divide the length of the book by 13 days. Tell your child he's going to do a little bit of the book reading and report each day and can earn some kind of reward he enjoys for completing each segment. This reward needs to be given right after the work is done. Now have your child read one-twelfth of the book each evening with you and jot down some notes. The child can even use doodles or other drawings instead of phrases or words. Believe it or not, we are more likely to remember things we draw, even simplistic doodles, than words or written descriptions. Now have the child compose several sentences about what he has just read from his notes. He can type this into a word processor or you can do it for him if he isn't yet fluent in using a word processor. Do this every day for 13 days and you have the raw material needed to make the book report. On the 14th day, you spend time that evening helping your child review, edit, spell-check, and otherwise polish his report. Now he's ready to turn in his report the next day.

Use 3" × 5" file cards for multistep projects. Write a step on each card and then put them in the sequence in which they are to be done. Write on the top of the card the day and time you and your child will go that step together. You can even write these steps on sticky notes instead and put each note on its appropriate day and time on a week-at-a-glance calendar. Either way, the task is broken down into steps, and a time is chosen for getting each step done. Keep this in a location that's easy for your child or teen (and you) to see and refer to it often as to when the next step will be done.

Break down shorter assignments that your child has trouble sticking with. Consider the nightly math assignment. Your child has been told to do 30 math problems on an assignment sheet. This is a large amount of work for a child with ADHD to do at one sitting. You can eliminate the child's timing disability here by simply doing what you did above for the book report. Have your child do just five or six problems. Give him a small reward or some points in a point or token system. Then let him have a brief break of a few minutes. Now have him do the next five or six problems. Again reward him and again give him a minute or two of break time. Keep at it, and in no time the entire assignment is done. But it was done in five or six sittings and not one (see the box below). Virtually any task that takes more than 5–10 minutes can be broken down this way to be more compatible with your child's ADHD and the 30% delay in executive age (EA) discussed in the chapter on Principle 3.

Create a daily timeline for school days. A timeline is a long sheet of paper (or many sheets taped together). For younger children, this can contain pictures of each routine activity the child does every weekday that are taped together into a sequence or chain. On each picture, at the top border, write the typical time period these things are done. For older kids,

What about *Your* Time?

Yes, breaking up tasks this way will make the whole assignment take a little longer than another child requires, and that means it will also take up your time. But it won't take as long as it normally would for an ADHD child, who is not likely to even do this assignment as originally structured without being implored repeatedly to get back to work, which of course doesn't succeed (see Principle 7). Also by breaking the task into smaller quotas, you keep the whole endeavor positive. You're helping your child gain competence and confidence, making him see that it's easily feasible to do the assignment, keeping him motivated with small rewards, and making the assignment as a whole feel less onerous. All of this adds up to a more positive relationship with your child.

this can just be a two-column list. The second column sets forth the activities for a typical day that can be subdivided into sections of the day. Next to each task or subdivision you can specify the usual times to do it in the first or lefthand column. You can hang this timeline in the child's room or in your kitchen. For instance, the following list includes the simple tasks the child must do on a typical school day:

- Wake up
- Wash up
- Get dressed
- Have breakfast
- Brush teeth
- Get bookbag (and lunch bag if needed)
- Get in car (or go to bus stop)
- Attend school (if the school day follows a routine, you can add it to this timeline)
- Have a snack after school
- Play
- Do homework
- Have dinner (or have dinner before homework)
- Watch TV or play games
- Read with Mom or Dad
- Brush teeth
- Undress and put PJs on
- Go to sleep

For older children, you could put just an after-school timeline in the kitchen that shows what chores or tasks the child is to do after school and during what time block. Put this shorter timeline where it is quite visible, such as on the refrigerator door or a cabinet door. You can also make a chore timeline for Saturday mornings and post it there.

Use a calendar to show your child how many days there are before some special activity or event (birthday, holiday, vacation, etc.). Remember, time moves really slowly when a child with ADHD is waiting for a future event to occur! Have your child mark off the days each morning so he can visually track how many days are left.

Manage Waiting Time: Distract Your Child with Activities

Speaking of waiting, there are times when waiting for something is inevitable and unavoidable, such as in waiting rooms for doctors' appointments, in lines to buy things, or when a child has to wait before going to do things she enjoys (going to a movie, etc.). What can you do to help your child wait?

Take along something diverting. In many modern families, parents have smartphones on which they can install fun video or word games for their child to play while waiting. Or take along a small toy that the child enjoys playing with that can help to pass the time.

For unanticipated waits, get creative and act fast. Even if you haven't brought such things with you, you can still try to think of things to do. All parents are used to digging into their bag for something to draw with when food takes too long to arrive at a restaurant. Or singing a song or playing a road trip game when traffic keeps you sitting in the car for too long. Use your imagination and your knowledge of what's diverting for your child, but do it before the child has a chance to get irritable or whiny.

WORKING MEMORY ISN'T WORKING

Offload It and Make It Physical!

> **THE PROBLEM:** Children with ADHD can't hold in mind the information they need to complete tasks.

The simplest definition of working memory is that it is remembering what to do. As noted in the Introduction, your child and others with ADHD have problems with this special kind of memory, which is something like the GPS in your car in that it's used to guide behavior toward a goal and toward the future in general. Like a GPS, this special memory uses images (hindsight and foresight) and words (self-instructions) that are being held actively in our mind to control our behavior toward a goal. But the child with ADHD seems less able to recall such images and instructions and especially to hold them in mind while working. And when any distraction shows up, what little working memory the child has gets erased. Without it, the child goes off aimlessly, doing whatever seems fun to do at the moment, like a car with a rogue GPS.

ADHD Is a Disorder of Doing What You Know, Not Knowing What to Do

This weakness in working memory has taught us something really important about ADHD: that it's a disorder of performance, not skill. In most cases, children with ADHD know what most other children their age know. But they can't use that knowledge to guide and control their behavior in specific situations where doing so would make a big positive difference in the outcome. Ten-year-old Josh tries to fly across a ditch on his skateboard and crashes to the pavement on his bare knees because he can't keep in mind that he's tried this before and fallen. After earlier attempts, he's realized that the ditch is 6 feet wide and he can't get enough speed going on the bumpy street to make it. But he can't turn that hindsight into foresight to prevent him from trying the same doomed trick over and over. Of course the inclination to act without thinking also means that even the first time he tried this leap he couldn't access his knowledge from prior skateboarding experiences or his natural ability to judge distances fast enough to pause and think better of it.

Unfortunately, those with ADHD also often avoid using hindsight to learn from their mistakes because it just feels too demoralizing to repeatedly acknowledge that they should have known better. So they usually just move on—to the next impulse.

Your Child Doesn't Lack Intelligence

The brain diagram on the facing page might help you understand that, in a very real sense, ADHD cleaves two parts of the brain from each other—the back half, where knowing occurs, and the front half, where doing occurs. Most children with ADHD don't have any problem with knowing. It's the fact that this knowledge doesn't show up in their behavior that makes many observers think they do. No wonder these kids are often demoralized and try to avoid feeling that way. Many people think that the way they act must mean they lack intelligence. On the contrary, children with ADHD know pretty much what other kids of the same age and community know! They have the same range of intellectual aptitudes that we see in the entire population.

Your Child Isn't "Bad"

If you often find yourself getting angry at your child with ADHD, it's probably because you know your child isn't stupid. So why *won't* she use the knowledge you know she has to do what's expected of her? Sadly, some parents and other authorities draw the conclusion that the child must simply be irresponsible, malicious, just plain "bad." That's why reminding

The Brain as a Knowledge versus Performance Device

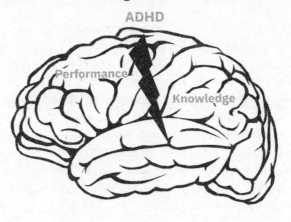

yourself that your child's behavior is not a matter of "won't" but of "can't" is so powerful in promoting a lasting positive relationship with your child—one that enables you to help your child to the full extent of your abilities. People with ADHD don't *choose* to act impulsively and so disregard what they know about how to behave in various situations. They have an inherent brain-based problem with working memory and impulse control.

You Can't "Fix" a Child with ADHD by Teaching Knowledge and Skills

Decades of research on skill training with children and teens with ADHD has shown that it doesn't work very well. And yet many teachers and professionals keep going down this road because they think that children with ADHD act as poorly as they do because they just don't know how to behave well. "Hey, if your son doesn't have friends and behaves poorly around other children, let's put him in a social skills group." "If your daughter is poorly organized or can't manage her time well, let's get her some remedial help with organizational skills." Makes sense on the face of it. But skills and knowledge aren't the real problem here. Using the skills *when* they are required, *where* it would be helpful is the problem. Can these children learn the skills? Yes. Do they need to be trained in these skills? Probably not. A refresher course in particular skills might be of minor help, but will they use those skills in situations where they should? Nope.

The bottom line here is that it's largely a waste of time and energy to try to teach children with ADHD information and skills that their brain can't easily access and employ in practice when and where it counts—when they would inform behavior. (This applies not just to how you try to help your child personally but also to therapies and special education methods—avoid the ones that focus solely on skill training and knowledge.) Instead, alter the point of performance to help them show what they know. The point of performance is that place in the natural environment where using that knowledge or set of skills would have been helpful. Modify that setting to prompt and cue your child and reward her for demonstrating and using that knowledge right there, right then. All effective parental help and all effective treatment takes place at *the point of performance*.

This advice applies to helping your child get around most of the executive function deficits of ADHD. When it comes to helping your child overcome a weak working memory in particular, the solution is straightforward: don't require your child to remember all of the knowledge and skills he needs or to keep them all in mind while working.

> **THE SOLUTION:** Offload working memory and make it physical.

Think about what your child needs to know or to remember when it comes to doing a particular task or assignment. And keep in mind that your child can't remember it and hold it in mind while working on the task at hand.

Transfer necessary information to a visible storage device outside your child's brain. Rather than demand that the child must remember this sort of information and keep it in mind, transfer the important information to a piece of paper or put it on sticky notes, file cards, or charts. Make it physical and put it where your child can see it when needed—that is, at the point of performance for that task. **Make lists.** When you routinely write a "to-do" list, this is precisely what you're doing—writing your ideas down (offloading them) on some other physical space (paper) so as to store and more easily recall them. You also place your list where you can see it often. All this helps you remember what you're supposed to be doing. We all benefit from some aids to working memory, but your child with ADHD really needs them. So try writing short, simple lists for your child about chores (see "Make chore cards" below), homework assignments, house rules, and anything else you want the child to keep in mind when she *can't* do it on her own—and put them where she'll need them and see them when that type of work has to get done. Put the house rules on the fridge, where the child will see them often and be reminded that they apply throughout your home. Put the before-school prep routine on your child's closet door or the back of the door through which the child departs for school (or both!). Put a list of washing-up steps or tooth-brushing steps (or both) on the bathroom mirror. Sticky notes were invented just for this purpose—to remind us of the tasks we need to remember to do where and when we'll be doing them. You can find lots of free chore lists broken down by age at the Focus on the Family website. WebMD also lists what chores are appropriate for a given age, while other websites provide charts that you can download to further organize chore lists. (See the Resources at the end of the book.) For a child with ADHD, you may need to break down each chore into its very specific steps.

Make picture sequences. This storing of information on some device doesn't just have to be in words or lists. Pictures can work just as well or even better and can be recalled more readily than verbal instructions. That is especially true for younger children or those who may have ASD along with ADHD. So when your child has something to do, you can not only write down the steps on a card and have the child keep it with him while working but also have him draw simple pictures of each step to make a picture sequence. You can also find many such picture sequences already created on the Internet, many of which are free, for most routine tasks children have to complete. Just google "picture sequences for children" and you will find lots of them. Even if they are aimed at children with ASD or intellectual disability, all children can benefit from picture sequences displayed at key locations where routine tasks are done, such as bathing, dressing, brushing teeth, washing hands, cleaning up bedrooms, and more. The important thing here is to use some physical cue to remind your child of what is to be done in this place at this time.

Provide written rules for work. Your child may be about to sit down and do homework at the kitchen table. What general steps should she follow? These steps might include:

1. Survey the task

2. Read the instructions

3. Then answer the first question

4. Write it down

5. Review it for accuracy

6. Then go to the next question

7. Repeat

Write these steps down on a card in the order in which they are to be done. It helps to add some kind of reward (see Principle 7) to the card for following the steps correctly and completing the assigned work. Then place this card in front of the child so he can refer to it while working. Obviously, this strategy, just like the list making above, requires that a child be old enough to read and comprehend the verbal rules written on the card. For younger children, see the picture sequence suggestion above.

Make chore cards. You can also do this for the routine chores you ask your child to do, like put toys away in the family room , pick up her room, load or empty a dishwasher, feed and pour water for the family pet, set the table for dinner. Each chore can have its own file card, and each card contains the steps the child is to follow in order to do that task (see Principle 7). Nearly all tasks a child has to do can be broken down into their simpler steps and then these steps written down on a card to keep in front of the child while she's working. For instance, for cleaning up a bedroom, a parent might list these steps:

■ Straighten up your bedding: Pull top sheet back up to top of bed. Then pull up your blanket or bedspread back to the top of your bed. Place your pillow at the head of your bed.

■ Pick up dirty clothes on the floor and bed, then place them in the clothes hamper or bin in your closet.

■ Put toys back in toy boxes, bins, or on shelves where you usually keep them.

- Pick up trash, uneaten food, food wrappers, and wastepaper and put them in your trash can.

- Take dirty dishes back to the kitchen and put them next to the sink.

Again, this strategy is for children who already can read and comprehend; for younger children, use picture reminders or even picture sequences (described above).

Encourage self-talk out loud. Another thing you can do to reinforce your child's working memory during a task is have him talk out loud to himself during the task about what he's supposed to be doing. He can read and recite the rules or steps you put on the file card to keep his mind on those rules or instructions. You can also prompt him while working to tell you what step he's doing and what the next step is. This keeps the child's mind focused on the work.

Self-talk is best for children older than 5 years of age. For younger children, self-speech has not yet acquired its ability to control or guide behavior. Instead, you may need to provide gentle periodic reminders to your child throughout the task being tackled.

Create behavior contracts. For older children and teens, it can be very helpful to both memory and motivation to create a behavior contract. Sit down with your child to discuss a particular task or goal she has trouble completing. Write a contract together that states what the task is, how often it is to be done, in how much time, and that it is to be done when requested. Then state in your contract what your child will earn for doing so. This can be money, points, tokens, time spent on a favorite activity such as electronic devices, and the like. The contract can contain only the reward to be earned or also what your child will lose if she doesn't perform the work as requested. This penalty works best if the child is on some sort of token or point system in which she is fined points for not doing the work (see Principle 7). Otherwise, you can start with just the reward portion of the consequences being stated in the contract and then add the punitive part if that is necessary later on. After the contract is written, have your child sign it, and you should too. Then post it in a visible place like the refrigerator door.

What about smart technology? Given how commonplace smart technology is in our lives and those of our children, it's very tempting to search for gadgets, apps, and websites that promise to organize your child, remind her of what needs to get done and how to do it, and, especially, when it should get done (time management aids). Some devices and apps for smartphones or tablets might be helpful just to give simple reminders of when something should be done, such as taking prescribed ADHD medicine at particular times of the day. Dr. Joseph Biederman and his colleagues have developed an app to assist with reminders for when to take medication and, especially, when the prescription needs to be refilled that is proving helpful to adults with ADHD and parents of children and teens with ADHD. But that is really not intended to help children directly. Another resource, the WatchMinder, may also prove helpful. It is a watch with a digital display that sends out simple reminders of when something needs to get done, such as getting to appointments or taking medication. (See the Resources at the end of the book.) These days smartphones have calendar apps with reminders that can serve this purpose just as well. You can find a variety of websites showing other apps for ADHD by just googling "apps + ADHD" in your browser. But in my clinical experience and that of many of my colleagues, these devices and apps are just not as effective as one would think for assisting with working memory and sense of timing for various reasons:

▪ Someone needs to make sure the device is charged and know where the device and cord are even located at the moment (people with ADHD are notorious for misplacing such things and forgetting to charge them).

▪ Someone has to initially find, buy, and install the app or device and then put the important information (dates, times, what is to be done, lists of other details, etc.) into it. The person with ADHD is unlikely to do so reliably or completely each week or whenever the calendar or list needs to be updated with new key information.

▪ The device needs to be with the child or teen when it reminds him of what to do and when to do it (and, as noted above, those with ADHD frequently forget to take the device along when they leave situations, whereas paper lists, cards, notes, and other cues are placed where they are needed so they can be seen instantly in that situation when that task needs to get done).

▪ The key information is out of sight, hidden as it is in the app or device until the moment the reminder is activated. (People with

ADHD benefit from things like lists or reminders being in and staying in their visual field so they can see them repeatedly even if it is not yet time to do the relevant task.)

For these and other reasons, low-tech paper aids, such as single-page lists, sticky notes, file cards, and week-at-a-glance calendars placed at key points in a child's environment—lying open on a desk or kitchen table or stuck on a refrigerator or other door—seem to work far better than smart technology and its apps.

Don't Overdo the Reminders!

In Principle 7, I cautioned you to watch for the possibility that rewards were being overused—that they were being applied to every single task the child was supposed to do, or the child was becoming more interested in the whole reward system than in the accomplishments that were being rewarded. The same caveat applies to offloading information to assist your child with working memory. You don't want to overwhelm your child with excessive detail and the unnecessary clutter of too many notes and reminders in places where work is to be done or an instruction obeyed. The external storage devices you use should include just enough information to remind the child of what she already knows and the basics of what is to be done. The goal is not to provide a skills manual or to teach the information from scratch. Single words or short phrases and/or picture cues or sequences can be just enough to trigger what the child already knows about what to do in a particular situation. I once got into the car of an adult with ADHD who was a sales rep for a drug company. I couldn't help noticing that his entire dashboard, including the gauges (!), was covered with sticky notes. He used these as reminders of things he needed to do or places he had to be at specific times, but there were probably a hundred of them! Talk about being distracted! The seven-step list for homework shown above exemplifies how simple and concise the language on your child's reminders should be. For further assistance in creating lists of chores and other reminders for children, just google "chore lists for children," and many websites will appear that offer various lists and charts by age.

GET ORGANIZED

I don't have to tell you that children with ADHD are disorganized. You're likely surrounded by the evidence of this particular executive function weakness. From the chaos of your child's bedroom to the backpack stuffed with crumpled paper and play areas that look like the proverbial bomb hit them, your child's home environment is in constant disarray. Your child's teachers know about this aspect of ADHD too: your child's "completed" assignments are missing pieces, books vanish, notes sent home for parents' signatures are never seen again. If you and your child's teachers have put reward systems in place (Principle 7), your child may be more motivated than in the past to get—and keep—his stuff together. If your child has been given point-of-performance reminders (Principle 9) about what to do with homework materials, his clothing, and his toys, you might no longer have to do all the cleanup all the time. If your child uses external clocks to substitute for his absent internal clock (Principle 8), maybe more of his assignments actually get finished these days. But getting organized will always be a struggle.

> **THE PROBLEM:** ADHD disrupts self-organization.

A major problem for people with ADHD is the difficulties they have with organizing things in their life so they can be more efficient, timely, and effective in meeting their daily responsibilities and other demands related to their work and life. Yes, we all suffer from disorganization periodically—such are the demands of life these days that it's hard to find the time to be and stay organized for maximum efficiency. But children and teens with ADHD take this to an entirely new level, placing as they often do in the bottom 7% of kids their age in their degree of organization.

Many of the executive function deficits described in the Introduction (not just the specific problem with organization, planning, and problem solving) conspire to create disorganization in people with ADHD.

Their mental filter is filled with holes. This problem with organizing things starts in the mind, where those with ADHD often describe their thinking as a jumbled mess. The human mind is designed to admit multiple ideas that enter our consciousness from everywhere so that it can put together all kinds of closely and vaguely associated ideas and form the resulting connections. When the mind is not being put in the service of accomplishing some goal or task, this mental bouncing around goes on unimpeded. When something does demand our focused attention, most of us can zero in on it, temporarily shutting out the irrelevant input. But in ADHD, it's much harder to shut down the mind's natural penchant for wandering. When your child with ADHD tries to think about tasks that must be done—and your child *does* try, even though you may find that hard to believe sometimes—other thoughts may creep in and distract her. Daydreaming takes over. And little mental work gets done.

Enter the working memory deficit . . . As you know from Principle 9, children with ADHD also find it difficult to hold information in mind while they consider ways to reach a goal.

. . . And the time management deficit. Principle 8 explained why your child struggles with time and time management. But it also helps us to understand why she finds it difficult to put the actions she is thinking of taking into the right or most efficient order for doing them. After all, time is really a sequence of events, so if you have trouble with the former you will also struggle with timing the sequence of things as well.

The general problems with attention and self-restraint tip the balance. If these problems weren't enough to make a child with ADHD disorganized, add in the fact that inattention and weak impulse control are enough to sidetrack your child by making it really hard for her to ignore distracting events that may be occurring around her. Those events are more compelling in capturing their attention and subsequent reactions than are the task-related things she was thinking about doing.

And without a strong capacity to self-motivate, organization

doesn't stand a chance. On top of these various difficulties, your child often won't have the level of motivation needed to organize his life. He'll seek shortcuts to getting things done while applying the least amount of effort possible (lack of persistence). It will feel much easier to drop things he's been using where he just used them than to put them back where they belong. So, it is not just the mind of a child with ADHD that is a mess but also her home, work space, school space, and life more generally. Organizing things and returning them to where they belong can take a little extra time and effort now even though they pay off in greater efficiencies later. But, alas, the "laters" in life are not in the immediate thoughts of someone with ADHD and thus are not compelling reasons to be and stay organized. That is why being organized is in such short supply when someone has ADHD.

THE SOLUTION: Help your child get and stay organized at the point of performance.

As with helping your child compensate for deficits in a sense of time and working memory, applying solutions right where a task needs to be done is key. So the first step in helping a child with ADHD get and stay organized is to survey where your child is currently *dis*organized and where being disorganized is having an adverse effect on his home, work, school, and/or social life. Where is the problem? Quickly catalog these places and spaces with your child and prioritize which ones need to get straightened up first. And in "point of performance" I'm including not only place but also time—the work periods when your child is having problems due to lack of organization.

Although each work space is different and may need to be organized differently for maximum efficiency, there are some general rules you can follow in organizing any workspace for your child:

WHERE is the work being done? Is this the best place to do it? Is it ADHD-friendly, with few if any distractions? Can that work place be supervised frequently by you or your child's teacher when the child is working there? If not, then change the location or rearrange it so it fulfills these requirements. For one child I know, the little alcove off the family room turned out to be a better homework space than the side of his bedroom where his parents had placed his desk. His room was filled with his toys, which were a constant distraction, and the family room was next to the kitchen, where his parents spent a lot of time. The alcove had been designated as Mom's office space, but she was happy to give it over to her son when she realized it had bookshelves and drawers for his materials and was right where she could check on him regularly while he worked.

WHAT materials need to be located here that are often used in getting this type of work done? Look at anyone's work, school, or homework desk and you should find the usual important materials, from pencils to blank paper, sticky notes, file cards, a ruler, a stapler, some tape, paper clips, maybe even a calculator, and usually some kind of lighting. Depending on your child's age, there might also be a computer or tablet. No matter the work, these materials and devices support our performance of many different tasks. Besides such things, people usually have a calendar that is opened to that day so they can see what work is due or what things need to be done. And they may also have a small lined writing pad on which is printed their "do" list for this project—the steps they need to follow to do that particular, often complex project. They've typically broken it down into smaller steps or work quotas (as described in preceding principles) to simplify the work and make it seem less insurmountable—and therefore more likely to get done.

What about your child's work spaces? Whether your child does her homework at the kitchen table or a dedicated desk somewhere else, are all these materials close at hand, maybe on a shelf in the kitchen or in cubbyholes over the desk? Don't think about just what you're seeing in the child's current work space but also what you often have to hunt down elsewhere because your child has misplaced it ("Mom, where are my scissors?"). You and your child can make a list of what should always be available for the task in each space. Here are some examples:

■ *Desk.* Paper, pens and pencils, art supplies, to-do list (an erasable board is nice) for homework, assignment book, reward record if you're using one (see Principle 7), timer if you're using one (see Principle 8), and so forth.

■ *Backpack.* Most parents would agree that the backpack a child takes to school every day should have its own special place (such as on a peg or shelf near the door the child exits through in the morning) and that everything that needs to go into it should either be in it already the night before or be organized at that spot. A checklist of what should be in it is helpful for last-minute reviews too.

■ *Sports equipment.* Children with ADHD need the outlet of exercise more than other kids, and yet they're the first ones to arrive at sports practices without some of their equipment. Can you assign a particular spot in the house for this stuff? If you drive your child to practice, is there a shelf in the garage where it can't be missed? A checklist of what your child needs to take to practice is great here too, or you could label slots on a shelf where each piece of gear should be stored.

■ *Bedroom.* A lot depends on your child's age, but have a system (with labels as working-memory aids) for storing clean clothes, dirty laundry, toys and books, and so on.

■ *School supplies.* Again, depending on your child's age, if you can do so it's often helpful to check out your child's classroom desk and/or locker to see if that needs to be organized as well. And for home use, make sure you have materials to help your child organize her work, such as notebooks, Trapper Keepers, color-coded upright filers and folders, an accordion folder, and pencil/pen stands, holders, or boxes.

WHEN is the best time for this kind of work to be done? At school, the work has to be done when class is in session and the teacher has assigned in-class work. But at home there is some flexibility. So, think about when your child is most likely to be willing (and able) to do the work required:

■ *Children with ADHD should usually not be asked to do homework as soon as they arrive home from school.* Their motivational batteries are exhausted from a full day of schoolwork and other demands on their self-regulation. Their executive fuel tank is low, and it needs refueling. Most parents would let their child have a snack after school, go play for a while, and so recharge their motivational batteries. Then the parent can require the child to do any school homework just before (or just after) dinner.

■ The best time for household chores, like cleaning up a

bedroom, is usually on the weekend and then before the child gets to do any leisure activities. Every child is different, of course, so think about your child's energy levels through the day and the week and when she usually has the strongest focus and schedule tasks accordingly. Maybe a brief, simple chore can be done after dinner and before playing or TV, but larger chores should wait for Saturday morning. Or maybe a large chore should be broken into segments to be done on weekdays because your child values putting all of her valuable resources into a sport or other activity on Saturdays.

Also, don't forget that children with ADHD may be as disorganized in their play spaces as their work spaces. There are lots of great videos and websites on the Internet on this topic. There are also products like toy shelves, storage bins, and other materials for getting their bedrooms and playrooms better organized and helping them to keep it that way.

Again, the idea of this chapter is not mainly to give you lots of specific things you can do to help organize your child's work and play life and spaces. There are plenty of ideas for those things on the Internet. The point of this chapter, like that of this book, is to educate you about the governing principles you need to keep in mind in taking charge of ADHD and why you need to know them. Once you know the why, the how is easier to see and implement. From those principles, the details flow and make perfect sense. But if you don't know the principles and the "why" behind them, then the details of what to do won't be nearly as obvious or as effective. And you surely won't explore your own inventive ideas about how to address the principles with your own child.

You also must remember that the child with ADHD has a disability and it leads him to have this high level of disorganization. And it will usually cause the child to return to it if not periodically monitored. That means you will have to supervise your child more closely and often while he's working, help to redirect him as needed, find ways to motivate him to stick with it, and periodically check his work spaces and other places to see that he stays organized. If they are not supervised in this way, over time children with ADHD often return to their chaotic and disorganized ways of doing things, as do their work places and play spaces.

Get Organized with the Help of the Internet!

Numerous websites and other online sources provide tips (and sell products) that can help you get your child with ADHD organized. They are listed in the Resources at the back of the book, but here is a list of organizational steps to take from *ADDitude* magazine (dedicated to ADHD).

IN THE BEDROOM

- Clear off the bed.
- Sort through the desk.
- Set up a clear spot for trash.
- Organize any bookshelves.
- Set up a reading spot.
- When in doubt, label it.
- Organize the "monsters" [the mess] under the bed.
- Store off-season clothes in bins or a separate section of the closet.
- Put laundry front and center.
- Categorize clothing.
- A week of shelves in the closet for a full week of outfits.
- Add shoe racks.

IN THE PLAYROOM

- Make a place for toys.
- Toss out old toys.
- Repurpose whenever possible.
- Create play centers.
- Make things double up.

IN THE CHILD'S WORK SPACE

- Use the walls.
- Get a planner.
- Make a master calendar.

- Make a school-only shelf.
- Tackle the backpack.
- Keep backpacks clean.
- Sort supplies.
- Make a map (of what goes where in the backpack).
- Ask for an extra set of school textbooks (to put in the home work space).
- Display your child's best work (at the work space).
- Designate a study space.
- Schedule a consistent homework time.

Note. From *www.addituedemag.com/organizing-kids-rooms*. Used by permission of Wayne Kalyn.

Don't Let the Organization Overtake Its Purpose

Too much focus on being organized can become hyperneatness and actually get in the way of efficiently accomplishing the work and other projects children need to get done. Too much time spent organizing is too little time spent actually getting the flow of work done in a reasonable time. Neatness in printing up folder labels, straightening up desk materials so that they are perfectly aligned, focusing on decor and its colors and patterns and being certain pencils are sharpened to a perfect point do nothing to facilitate productivity. Instead they put the focus on the aids to getting the work done instead of the work itself.

Also, studies show that being a bit impulsive and disorganized may contribute to creativity. That's because it allows individuals to explore novel ways of combining ideas or parts of a project that more organized and obsessively goal-directed people would not have noticed. They would actually have unconsciously or consciously inhibited such unusual mental associations to stay focused on the goal—and pared away too much of the other input and associations that the mind makes. Obviously, identifying the appropriate line between staying focused on the goal and letting the imagination have enough freedom to come up with innovations is not always easy. For parents of children with ADHD the key to finding this demarcation line is to pay close attention to how their child works and thinks and what emerges. See Principle 5 for reminders about staying aware.

And even when promoting creativity is not your goal, find times during your child's work to encourage her to let loose and have some fun with the materials she has and the ideas that flow through her naturally inventive mind. This kind of break can rejuvenate both of you. And it can go a long way toward easing frustration and stress when your patience with the mess around you has been stretched to its limit.

MAKE PROBLEM
SOLVING CONCRETE

As familiar as you are with your child's penchant for disorganization (Principle 10), you're also well acquainted with problems your child has with problem solving. Maybe your 6-year-old son gets frustrated when he can't have all the flavors of ice cream because he can't seem to pick one favorite. Or your 8-year-old daughter has trouble making friends because she doesn't know how to compromise when a group of kids all want to play make-believe differently. Many parents have told me about their children who are constantly getting hurt because they can't assess the risks involved in following their energetic impulses and choose actions that protect their own safety.

Besides physical harm, a weakness in problem solving often produces an emotional meltdown because the child has to suffer the consequences of making poor choices—or even of making no choice at all. As a parent you may sympathize with your child's disappointment but not with the fact that your child keeps making bad decisions, despite all of your coaching, skill training, and knowledge dispensing. As you know if you've read the preceding principles, all the knowledge and skill in the world isn't going to erase your child's ADHD-related executive function deficits. But that doesn't mean there's nothing you can do to help your son or daughter with a weakness in problem solving. Principles 2–4 hopefully have helped you adopt a compassionate attitude and a deeper understanding of the fact that your child's frustrating behaviors stem from a neurological problem. It's not "won't" but rather "can't." This can go a long way toward preventing frustrating failures to problem-solve from driving a wedge between you and your child.

But, of course, that won't necessarily help your child problem-solve where and when he needs to do so. That's what the rest of this chapter is about. And in Principle 12 you'll find help with preventing the emotional meltdowns that stem from a weakness in emotion regulation skills—not by teaching new skills but by planning and tweaking the environment in which the meltdowns often occur to lessen their frequency.

Problem solving is required in all realms of daily life and with increasing sophistication as children grow. Even an infant is doing a very primitive sort of problem solving when she cries and then cries louder when no parent responds right away. A very young child is engaging in problem solving when he figures out what he can build with the blocks or Legos he has. A child in elementary school is literally solving problems when she does her math homework. When your child is approaching adolescence, he has to start doing complex problem solving to figure out how to do what he wants to while observing the laws of his community, meeting the expectations of family, and trying to achieve his personal goals. But the critical function of problem solving is even harder than getting organized for a person with ADHD, especially when it must be done in their mind.

> **THE PROBLEM:** People with ADHD have trouble holding things in mind and manipulating them to solve problems.

You and I call it problem solving. Children call it play. When children play, they begin by taking things apart with their hands (manually). This is actually what we know as *analysis*. It allows children to see what parts are involved (in a toy, a puzzle, a tool or simple machine) and how they operate together to perform their function.

Eventually they will play with recombining these pieces in various ways, which is called *synthesis*. Young children play with actual puzzle pieces or blocks, testing out various combinations to see how they fit together to help create a structure or picture. Most of the combinations aren't very useful, but some unique ones can help a child build a Lego structure or complete a picture puzzle.

Through this process of analysis and synthesis, children learn about their world—that it can be taken apart, and that the resulting parts can be recombined in novel ways. It's a process we follow throughout life. Everything we take apart to understand how it works teaches us something about the individual components, and we use that understanding to put things back together. By the time we're adults, we have quite a store of information to use in problem solving.

Children start out doing this analysis and synthesis manually, but as they mature, they develop the mental capacity for visual imagery, which allows them to skip the manual manipulation and start moving around images in their heads. A child of age 4 or 5 might, for example, be able to hold some images in mind. We know this because drawing anything from memory requires that you have stored an image of what you are drawing in your mind and then activate that image to serve as the template for the drawing. But children this age are not yet able to take apart and recombine those images in their mind to create new ideas. That comes a few years later, and certainly by adolescence. Because the child has manipulated objects manually many times during earlier development, he eventually doesn't need to test out different combinations by moving the objects around; rather, he can call up images of moving them and efficiently move them on the first try to produce the desired results. He has found combinations he likes by doing the manual work, and now those favored combinations will be the first ones he applies when he encounters a similar problem. As they mature, children can play mentally with the elements of more and more problems they encounter until they find some combination that seems to solve the problem. They have now moved on from manual to largely mental play and problem solving.

The next step in the development of problem-solving capacity is to manipulate not just mental pictures but also words that represent problems we need to solve. Our problems don't involve only objects that we have to manipulate—unclogging a drain, sewing on a button, reorganizing a closet. We also need to manipulate words in our heads to decide what to write or say in a given situation.

Kids don't necessarily know consciously that they are trying to learn through analysis and synthesis so that they can store a treasure trove of options for various needs in their working memory. They do it just because it's inherently fun to do.

Typical children will analyze and synthesize instinctively as they become mobile and interact with their environment. So will children with ADHD. But as you'll recall from the Introduction, those with ADHD are behind in their development of executive functions. Unfortunately, this means they don't use visual imagery or manipulate words in their minds as early as typical children. And when they eventually do develop these mental abilities, they are bound to be less proficient at them than typical children. It also means that they are hampered by their executive function deficits in carrying out the steps of solving any given problem:

Children with ADHD have trouble holding information in mind to guide behavior toward a goal. Holding information in mind—working memory—is the foundation of problem solving. Imagine trying to accomplish even the simplest task—from wrapping a gift to making coffee to getting dressed—if you couldn't remember the steps that worked to solve the "problem" the last time you did it or how any required tools worked. You might end up with a package sloppily covered in tape and still not secured, coffee that is too weak or too strong, or rumpled clothing that doesn't go together.

Children with ADHD can't analyze and synthesize information as well as other children. Obviously if they can't keep the information they need in their mind and focus on it, they cannot take it apart or otherwise play with it to see if they can think up a way to solve the problem or accomplish the task they are doing. As I noted earlier, kids with ADHD often experience their minds as a "jumbled mess"—like a pile of puzzle pieces that don't seem likely to fit together in any way at all. Lacking the ability to mentally simulate problems and their solutions through analysis and synthesis, they're forced to resort to manually trying out various solutions—a slow, frustrating, and often unsuccessful way to deal with life's problems.

Children with ADHD cannot mentally manipulate words as well as typical children. As you know from living with a child who has ADHD, this is another weak area for those with this neurological disorder. They often don't write clearly (causing problems with school assignments), and they tend to blurt out inappropriate statements or questions that cause trouble in all sorts of interactions, resulting in social problems as well. A problem presented in verbal form often stops them in their tracks as they struggle to relate the words to a visual image and the visual image to tangible objects—and end up with a jumbled mess.

As a result, they seem to repeat the same trial-and-error behavior without learning from it. A child with ADHD will try the same daredevil trick and get injured every time—and still keep at it. Working on a math problem, the child might start from step one even after doing a hundred such problems, never assimilating the problem-solving process to get to the right answer efficiently (or at all, and always get stuck on the same mistake). The child might get reprimanded over and over by a teacher for pushing to the head of a line or noisily insisting on shouting out an answer to the teacher's question without raising her hand. All of these instances of not learning from mistakes come from a limited ability to analyze, synthesize, hold information in mind, and manipulate components of a problem to consider the available options.

Think about times when you've contemplated rearranging the furniture in a room. You don't keep physically moving things around until you find what you like; typically, people visualize in their mind the different pieces of furniture in different places. Then if they think one idea might work, they may actually move the furniture to that location. Notice how much time and effort contemplating different arrangements in our mind's eye can save us! We can simulate the environment in our mind and play with that simulation instead of with the physical environment itself, sparing ourselves all the physical labor that would entail.

This ability not only saves us a lot of time and effort but also saves us from mistakes. That is because we can see in our mind how an error might occur and avoid it in real life. As the philosopher Karl Popper once said about this incredible capacity humans have for mental simulation, we can let our ideas die in our place. If we only learned by trial and error in the real world, as nearly all other creatures do, our mistakes could harm or even kill us. Mentally simulating events before we act is part of what we mean by contemplation. It is trial-and-error learning in our minds and not in real life, and it can not only lead to new solutions to old problems but save us from a lot of harm. Of course, people can do this type of play with words and phrases in their minds, not only with mental images. We can play around with what we want to say or write in our mind's voice to choose the best combination before we actually say or write something. I have done this quite a lot in writing this book, for instance.

And then there's distraction. Even when children with ADHD manage to hold information in working memory and consider the options for solving a particular problem, there's always a chance that something more interesting will distract the child and derail the sequence of mental steps needed to reach the solution.

Children with ADHD get distracted quite easily, and when they do, they lose that mental information and have to start over. They can't keep their mind focused on the problem long enough to solve it. Then they either have to start over in their thinking or just quit trying to solve that problem and go on to do something more fun and interesting. They are stuck back at the earlier, less mature stage of manually playing with their environment. While that is a necessary stage in developing mental problem solving, as I noted above, it's not very efficient compared to the later, more mature form of mental problem solving.

So how can we help children with ADHD do this kind of mental problem solving? It's important to do so because they will need to rely more and more on this mental ability as they grow up, in schoolwork and later in their jobs.

THE SOLUTION: Make problem solving physical and manual.

If your child is about 30% behind in the development of executive functioning, as I've said earlier, he's likely to still be trying to solve problems with his hands and not in his head. Even if your child is beginning to develop working memory and mental problem-solving abilities, his success can be enhanced by letting him also work on a problem with his hands. Your goal is to give your child the time to develop mental problem-solving abilities without becoming so discouraged that he gives up. The key is to allow him to succeed by using what he can already do— manipulate the parts of the problem manually.

Let's assume your child has some arithmetic homework to do, or a paragraph or two to write for English class. Can you think of a way to make the relevant pieces of the problem physical, as in a picture puzzle? Can you make it external and thus possible to manipulate manually? Or can you think of physical objects your child could use to represent the elements of the problem and manipulate them to assist in solving this type of problem?

Here are some ways to externalize arithmetic problems:

■ Give the child a number line, like a yardstick, on his desk. The child could then add and subtract simple numbers by just counting backward and forward along the number line. And if he's learning negative numbers as well, you can put two number lines or yard-sticks together so that at the center point is a zero and to the left of it are written in sequence the negative numbers of −1 to −20, for example, from the center going to the left.

▪ Give the child some poker chips, marbles, or Lego blocks and let her use her hands to count out the initial number of chips in the addition or subtraction problem that represents the first number in the math problem. Then the child could add or subtract the second number of chips to get the answer. This is often how we initially teach math to children—as something physical involving individual things in groups.

▪ Allow the child to use a calculator. This tool would make this entire operation easier, but teachers prefer that children learn the operation, such as addition or subtraction, before resorting to a calculator as a shortcut.

▪ Let the child work the problem out on a sheet of paper.

▪ Put in front of the child a table of numbers that looks like a matrix with the numbers 1–10 across the top and 1–10 down the left side. In each cell is the result of adding, subtracting, or multiplying the two numbers that converge there (the number at the top and the one at the far left). Now the child can go across and down the table to help him find the answers (and memorize the results).

What about the writing assignment? Let's say your child has to read a short story or chapter and write a brief essay about it. To make language manual and concrete, you could try the following.

▪ Have the child scan the entire story first. Just look at the material and what is on the pages (words, pictures, etc.).

▪ Then have the child read just the first paragraph or a short section.

▪ Now have her vocalize out loud what she just read about. You can prompt her thinking further by having a card in front of you with the questions "Who? What? Why? Where? When? How?"

▪ Then have the child write down some of her ideas or even just the answers to those questions. She can use a few words or a phrase or even draw (doodle) a simple picture if that helps. Nothing needs to be elaborate. The point is just to help jog her memory of what was important in that paragraph.

■ Now have the child review what she wrote to cement it more thoroughly in her memory of the story.

■ Then go on and have the child read the next paragraph and do the same things.

Read, recite, write, review. Notice that the child has now been exposed to the material about four times, which can help with retaining it. He has also learned to question himself about the content using those common single-word questions we all learned to use in this way. Also, notice that we not only had the child manualize or externalize the content by writing down some notes (or making some simple pictures); we had him vocalize it as well. That is another way of making information external and physical in its form—by saying it out loud. As I noted in the chapter on working memory, saying out loud the things we are trying to remember to do while we are doing them can reinforce our working memory of our goals and how we wanted to reach them, and it can keep us moving toward our goal.

Now once the short story has been read, your child can look at her notes and use that information to write some sentences about the story. She can start by writing down a sentence on what happened first, then a sentence on what happened next, and so on as she moves down her page of notes. Older children can even type these sentences about the story into a word processing program on a computer, which is another way of making the information physical in form. Now the child can manipulate what is in the document by editing, expanding, copying, pasting, and otherwise moving the contents around to make it read better. And the program can help spell-check the words and even suggest other words to use through its thesaurus menu option. Finally, have the child write a sentence or two on what she thought about this story, what she liked or didn't like about it, or how it made her feel. In other words, she can evaluate the story.

Four Steps to Every Solution

When faced with any sort of problem to solve, there are some general strategies that children can be taught to employ to help them along.

Step 1. State the Problem Out Loud.

What is the child being asked to do or think about? *For example:* Clean up his room.

Step 2. Break It Down.

Can it be specified in smaller steps? *For example:*

- Put away toys.
- Pick up any dirty laundry and put it in the hamper.
- Make the bed.

Step 3. Brainstorm!

Encourage your child to think and freely associate to the elements of the problem. What ideas pop into your child's head as he thinks about the nature of this problem? For kids with ADHD, be sure they (or you) **write each idea down** on a sticky note or 3" × 5" file card. Freely associated ideas are kind of like flying ducks or butterflies—you need to catch them as they fly by or they will fly right out of your mind and be hard or impossible to get back again. This is where the child with ADHD is at a great disadvantage—he can't hold his ideas in mind. So don't ask him to try. Get them down as soon as he (or you) can. Remember Principle 9 about working memory—offload it onto another storage device.

> *For example:*

- I want to use my Captain America costume later, so I'm going to leave it out.
- I can wear those PJs a couple more times, so I'll just put them on the bed instead of in the hamper.
- My sister Lisa was playing with the toy horses in here, so she should be the one to put those away.
- I can clean up my room later, after I finish the game I started.

While brainstorming with your child, never criticize the results, no matter how far-fetched, silly, ridiculous, or insane the idea is. The object, after all, is to get as much content out of the mind as possible. The ideas in the example may not be where you want to end up, but remember Principle 4—you can let some things go, like a perfectly made bed or a room cleaned up to your standards by 9 A.M. Saturday. Each brainstormed idea can be evaluated at the next step. But you can kill creativity and brainstorming by critiquing as you go. Perfectionistic children (rarely the problem in those with ADHD) or kids with low self-esteem (somewhat more common in ADHD) are likely to do this to themselves while brainstorming. So encourage them to shut down the critic in their mind and just free-associate to the problem and its elements. In short, get crazy and have some fun with this step even if all it does is make you both laugh about how silly and impractical some of the ideas can be.

Step 4. Critique and Sort the Ideas You Wrote Down.

Help your child decide which brainstormed ideas seem to help with the problem and which ones seem less helpful or even irrelevant. In critiquing each idea, follow this sequence:

- First have the child **state the advantages** of each idea and what she likes about it.
- Then have her think about and **state its disadvantages**, limitations, or impracticalities.
- Now your child can **organize** the ones that are helpful into a plan and **test it out** to try to see if it solves the problem they were given.

Think of this as the SOAPS method:

State the situation and break it down.

List the **O**ptions.

Note the **A**dvantages. Then note the disadvantages or **P**roblems with each.

Then see if a **S**olution is evident.

For example:

■ I want to use my computer game (tablet) later, but it may need to be charged up, so I'm going to plug it in while I play with it now, then leave it there on the counter to charge while I do something else, like have my dinner.

   ● Advantages: I won't have to wait for the game to charge up the next time I want to play with it—it will already be charged.

   ● Disadvantages: If I don't do this, my game will be dead and won't be charged up at all when I want to play with it, and I will be mad. But if I leave it on the counter and plugged in to charge, it might get in Mom's way when she starts cooking dinner. In that case, I will play with it and plug it in over on the sofa and just keep it there charging when I am not playing on it.

■ I can wear those PJs a couple more times, so I'll just put them on the bed instead of in the hamper.

   ● Advantages: The PJs will be where I'll be using them.

   ● Disadvantages: My bed will be messy, and it will be hard to make the bed with stuff on it.

■ Lisa, my sister, was playing with the toy horses in here, so she should be the one to put those away.

   ● Advantages: I won't have to do Lisa's cleanup, and all the toys will get put away.

   ● Disadvantages: Lisa will get in my way since I like to clean up fast and she doesn't. She probably won't put the horses back in the right place either. I'll have to clean up my room when she's available to do her part.

■ I can clean up my room later, after I finish the game I started.

   ● Advantages: I won't be tempted to stop cleaning up and go back to playing.

   ● Disadvantages: I don't know when I'll be finished with the game; it's a new one, so I'll probably just want to play it forever. That means my room will stay messy, and Mom will be mad.

   ● Solution: Putting off the room cleaning and leaving some things out instead of putting them away won't work. The job will never get done, and Mom and I will end up fighting about it all day. Here's what I'll do:

- I should keep my tablet plugged in while I play with it on the sofa so it isn't in anyone's way while they are working and it will keep charging even when I am not playing it.

- I should put my dirty clothes in the hamper first, because if I start putting my toys away first I might get distracted by wanting to play with them.

- There are toys all over my bed, so I have to put my toys away before I can make the bed.

- To stop myself from playing with the toys instead of getting them off the bed and stored away where they belong, I'll let myself keep one toy back and give myself 5 minutes to play with it before I make the bed.

- I'll ask Mom to set the timer for me just so I'll know when it's time to put that toy away and start making the bed.

- I don't have to make the bed perfectly, just as neatly as I can.

Notice that this child has tried to do his part to reduce potential conflict over both his play with his tablet and the chore of cleaning up his room (by recognizing that procrastinating and doing half of the job would aggravate Mom as would leaving his tablet on the kitchen counter) and that he and Mom have obviously gotten used to some compromising. If you need a refresher on these valuable strategies, go back to Principles 4–6 on setting priorities (letting go of the perfectly made bed standard), being there and aware, and helping your child become accountable, and Principle 8, making time real.

Other Problems to Solve by Making Them Manual, Concrete, or External

Social problems. Children with ADHD often have problems with making and keeping friends (their impulsiveness, hyperactivity, disorganization, and poorly regulated emotions can be challenging for others). You can use the SOAPS method to look at various options for all kinds of social problems:

- ■ Behaving appropriately on a play date or at a party
- ■ Sharing with siblings and classmates
- ■ Being a good sport on a team or in a group game
- ■ Following the house rules of relatives at holiday celebrations
- ■ Behaving appropriately at restaurants, religious services, movies, and live performances
- ■ Interacting with strangers

You can simulate many social problems by role-playing with your child. You are pretending to enact the social situation your child is having trouble with and test out or play with different ways of acting so your child or teen can see how they would turn out.

Self-help and self-care skills. You can use SOAPS, and in some cases role playing, to solve problems with dressing, bathing, brushing teeth, and more.

Handling responsibilities independently. The same is true for getting to the bus on time, getting homework done, meeting a teen's curfew, doing specific chores, and so forth. Each can be broken down into pieces or steps in a sequence and then put together to form a plan of action. Writing down each step or creating a picture of it is one way of making the steps of a problem physical and thus easier to remember and manipulate to make the right sequence for a plan of action.

Ideas for Making Mental Problems Manual and Physical

There are many clever ways to make mental problems manual and physical in some way so that your child with ADHD can work on them with her hands (and voice) and not just with her mind. Sometimes searching the Internet for pictures or picture sequences can give you ideas about how to do this for a particular kind of problem. Just writing down the parts of the problem can also help your child see and think about them better. See the Resources at the back of the book for more ideas.

BE PROACTIVE

Plan for Difficult Situations at Home and Away

Living with a child with ADHD can seem overwhelming or at least stressful much of the time. In the span of a single hour your child might go from getting into things she shouldn't at home to annoying her siblings to engaging in risky activities. Parents I've met in my clinical practice have told me their children got into the toxic cleaning products under the kitchen sink, the power tools in the garage, and the parents' medicine cabinet. They reported arguments with brothers and sisters over toys or what to watch on TV and lots of pushing and shoving or one-sided roughhousing. I heard their stories of kids trying to jump their bike off a homemade ramp in the driveway, climbing up on top of the frame of a swing set, crawling out onto a second-story roof from their bedroom window, pushing a kitchen knife into an electric socket, skateboarding into traffic, using sharp-edged can lids or power-saw blades as frisbees, and literally playing with fire. Children with ADHD have been known to go well beyond the developmentally healthy exploratory play described in Principle 11 that is a foundation for problem solving and experiment with pouring chocolate sauce on computers or TVs, pouring bleach into a clothes hamper, combining all of Mom's cosmetics on the bedroom carpet, smashing furniture with a hammer, feeding the dog socks, hanging the family cat out a window by its tail, and drawing on an expensive white SUV with a permanent marker—all just to see what would happen. Based on such parental reports, ADHD creates more stress within a family than nearly any other child psychological disorder, including autism.

Because they have so little self-control, children and teens with ADHD often require more "other control." Others have to step in to help manage their behavior when they seem unable to do so on their own as might be expected for a child their age. Of course, this task largely falls to you, the parent. You might feel like a firefighter, spending much of your time rushing from fire to fire, trying to put out the flames of your child's problem behavior. You may find yourself just waiting for that next problem to emerge, as you know it will, while trying to catch your breath and recover emotionally between these frequent behavioral conflagrations.

Interestingly, the problem here isn't really your child's lack of self-control—that's just a part of ADHD and something the child can't help. The problem is how you react to it.

THE PROBLEM: Parents of children with ADHD often operate in reactive mode.

Although they try to educate the public on fire prevention, firefighters generally can't help being in reactive mode. They can't anticipate a fire and head it off; they simply respond to the emergency call to put it out. Even though you may feel you're always doing damage control, the same is not really true for you. When you're rushing from one crisis to the next, you get into a mode of parenting that is mostly reactive—waiting for things to happen and then responding to them when they do. It's exhausting, and it doesn't really get you—or your child or the relationship between you—anywhere. Fortunately, there's an alternative to reactive mode.

THE SOLUTION: Get proactive!

To be proactive is to think ahead, plan for a problem situation, and implement your plan ahead of that situation in hopes that it will reduce or eliminate the problem. In Principle 4, you got some practice dealing with certain situations or settings beforehand to greatly diminish or even eliminate problems associated with them. In that chapter we focused on typical times of day or daily routines that can cause problems. You identified those time periods, mostly at home, that were ending in conflict between you and your child with ADHD because you were fighting over what the child had to do, how, and when. The main solution offered in that chapter was to prioritize the to-do list for that time period and cut down on the number of demands placed on your child. If you've put that principle into practice, you may already have reduced stress associated with routines like getting ready for school, doing homework, doing weekend chores, or getting ready for bed. But those regular daily or weekly routines aren't the only trouble spots for kids with ADHD. There are also all the places you have to go away from home—shopping, restaurants, relatives' and friends' houses—as well as rarer but predictable events at your own house, like holiday dinners you're hosting or your child's birthday parties.

What to do? The following strategies mostly target problem situations away from home, but you can also use them with daily routines, in addition to the prioritizing you did guided by Principle 4.

Make a list of problem situations, either at home or in public places. When time permits, perhaps in the evening after your child with ADHD has gone to bed, sit down and make a list of recurring problem situations. Where are these problems most likely to happen? If, despite your prioritizing, you're still having problems with certain events at home—when you have visitors, when you are on the phone, at homework time, at bedtime, when your child is asked to do a chore, or just during free time—write them down. Also consider places and events away from home—stores, restaurants, your house of worship, parks and playgrounds, the homes of relatives and friends.

Pick one problem situation and think about what typically happens. What usually happens in that situation? Take shopping in a grocery store, for instance:

■ When you enter the store, is the child off and running, down the aisles and away from you?

■ Is your child touching everything in sight? Putting things into your basket that you don't want?

■ Is the child demanding that you buy him something to eat or a toy he just saw on a counter or shelf? (Why do you think stores put candy and other attractive items at the checkout lane?)

Think of things you could do before or in the situation to head off the problem behavior. Now that you understand what is happening, think about whether some of the other principles in this book might help.

■ You could start by remembering that your child's EA (which might be age 6), is about 30% behind his chronological age (which might be 9), and asking yourself whether you should have even taken the child on this shopping trip to buy yourself clothing or cosmetics or groceries. Should you be taking a 6-year-old into a women's clothing store given how boring that will be for the child? Why not just line up a babysitter so you can shop in peace?

■ Maybe you could consider Principle 2 and remind yourself that your child has a disorder. His lack of self-control in this store isn't intentional; it's part of ADHD. You can change how you react, and you can plan ahead to head off some of the problem behavior, but that's about it. Accept that reality and some of your stress will subside before you enter a store, leaving you with greater resources to handle a shopping trip.

■ When you're in a store, prioritize per Principle 4—determine what you really have to get done and be prepared to gather and buy only the essentials if things don't go well. Think about how you might lower your standards for your child's behavior in the store to reduce conflict and get the errand done as quickly and calmly as possible.

■ Remembering Principle 8 and considering your child's time blindness and impatience, set the digital timer on your smartphone (the stopwatch function) when you enter a store and hand it to your child so he can see the time elapsing while you shop and he understands that this activity won't last long; seeing some of the time pass will make it easier for your child to wait till the end. Or, better yet, use better time management yourself—if you were shopping for groceries, can you order what you need online from that store and then set a pickup time to drive up to the designated parking spot and get your already bagged and paid-for groceries quickly?

■ Using what you learned in Principle 7, when you are shopping, pay attention to your child instead of just your grocery list, remind your child of how he is to behave, and get his attention with gentle touches.

Develop a transition plan. A transition plan is a set of steps you will take just before you enter or transition into that problem situation. To create one, you need to decide on the following:

■ *The rules.* Keep it to two or three rules you expect your child to obey in this upcoming situation. For example, if you're going into a store, tell your child (1) to stay near you, (2) not to touch anything without asking, and (3) not to ask you to buy anything.

■ *The reward.* What can your child earn for following the rules you have laid down? Do you plan to use a token system and give the child chips while shopping that she can use to buy something at the end of the trip (candy, ice cream, cheeseburger, etc.)? Or take her somewhere she enjoys right afterward? In short, what is your incentive to get the child to follow your rules?

■ *The punishment.* What do you plan to do for discipline if your child breaks a rule or otherwise misbehaves? Will you take away tokens? Put the child in a time-out location in a quiet corner of a store? (See the boxes on pages 162–163 and 164.) Take away some privilege?

■ *Something for your child to do.* Busy hands are happy hands when those hands belong to a child with ADHD. Here are some ideas you might consider for different problem situations:

● *For shopping,* take along something for your child to play with, such as a video game, your cell phone with a game installed on it, a Transformer toy or My Little Pony, or whatever your child likes to manipulate with his hands.

● Ask the child to get specific items off the shelf and place them in your cart.

● You can put a young child in the cart to contain her while shopping, but be sure she has something to do there. Some grocery stores even have shopping carts designed with small cars the child can ride in just beneath or in front of the cart.

- *At home,* think about what your child could be actively doing that will head off the problems you usually have. This may mean letting him help you with your task. Instead of leaving the child to his own devices while you go about your chores, which gives him ample freedom to misbehave, could you ask him to help you? Or could you ask him to do something he enjoys alongside you while you work, such as drawing, coloring, playing with clay, or building something with blocks?

- *If you are working outdoors,* could he play with a rake and try to rake leaves? Have a small garden spade to dig with in the dirt? Have a jar to collect particular insects that are around that time of year? Draw in chalk (washable) on the patio or driveway while you work outside? Physical activity decreases symptoms of ADHD for a short while and certainly keeps the child out of trouble. So have your child do something as simple as exercises, running around the outside of the house to a timer, playing hopscotch in the driveway, and the like.

Put the transition plan into action. Follow these steps before and during the problem situation:

■ *Stop!* Before entering any potential problem situation, stop and make sure you have explained your plan to your child. For instance, when going to the store, stop just outside the front door to go over your transition plan. *Never touch the door handle to a store without a plan.*

■ *Review.* Briefly state the rules you've come up with. If your child can read, consider having these written on a 3" × 5" file card that you can hand to the child to carry throughout that situation. If you're using the three rules for a shopping trip listed above, you could say even more simply, "Stand close, don't touch, don't beg."

■ *Repeat.* Have your child repeat your rules.

■ *Explain the reward.* Tell your child what she can earn, repeating it to remind her of the incentive to behave appropriately throughout the situation.

Using Time-Out in Public Places

Don't be afraid to use time-out in a public place, as it is the most effective method for teaching the child to obey rules in such places. After you've explained the punishment to the child, and immediately upon entering the public place, look around for a convenient time-out location in case you need one.

Here are some convenient time-out places:

IN DEPARTMENT STORES

- Take the child to an aisle that is not used much by others and place him facing a dull side of a display counter or a corner.
- Or take the child to the coat section and have him face the coat rack.
- Use a dull corner in the gift wrap/credit department area or a dull corner of a restroom.
- Use a changing or dressing room if nearby.
- Use a maternity section (these are usually not very busy and there are sympathetic moms there).

IN GROCERY STORES

- Have the child face the side of a frozen foods counter.
- Take the child to the furthest corner of the store.
- Find the greeting card display and have the child face the dull side of the counter while you look at cards.
- It is difficult to find a time-out place in most grocery stores, so you may have to use one of the alternatives to time-out listed in the box on page 164.

IN A HOUSE OF WORSHIP

- Take the child to the "crying room" found in most churches, where mothers take irritable babies during the service.
- Use the foyer or entryway to the church.
- Use a restroom off the lobby.

IN A RESTAURANT

■ Use the restrooms.

■ Otherwise, use one of the alternatives listed in the box on page 164.

IN SOMEONE ELSE'S HOME

Be sure to explain to your hosts that you are using a new child management method and you may need to place your child in a chair or stand the child in a dull corner somewhere if misbehavior develops. Ask them where one could be used. If this cannot be done, then use one of the alternatives listed in the box on page 164.

DURING A LONG CAR TRIP

Review the rules with the child and set up your incentive before having the child enter the car. Be sure to take along games or activities for the child to do during the trip. If you need to punish the child, pull off the road to a safe stopping area and have the child serve the time-out on the floor of the backseat or seated outside the car on a floor mat near the car. Never leave the child in the car unattended and never leave your child unsupervised if he is sitting outside the car.

If you use time-out in a public place, the minimum sentence needs to be only one-half what it normally is at home, because time-out in public places is very effective with children. Also, if the child leaves time-out without permission, take away some of the tokens or points that are part of her token system (see Principle 7).

■ *Explain the punishment.* Whatever you plan to do, tell the child up front—for example, before you enter a store.

■ *Give the child something to do right away.* Don't wait to provide this diversion. For example, you can give it to your child as soon as you enter a store.

■ *Give frequent feedback and rewards throughout the situation.* Don't be like most parents, who wait until the very end of a shopping

If You Cannot Use Time-Out
in a Public Place

There are always a few places where placing your child in a corner for misbehavior is not possible. Here are some alternatives, but they should be used only where you cannot find a time-out area:

1. Take the child outside the building and have him face the wall.

2. Take the child back to your car and have her sit on the floor of the backseat. Stay beside the child or in the front seat of the car.

3. Take along a small spiral notepad. Before entering the public place, tell the child that you will write down any episode of misbehavior and the child will then have to go to time-out for any misbehavior as soon as you get home. You will find it helpful to take a picture of the child when he is in time-out at home and keep this with your notepad. Show this picture to the child in front of the public place and explain that this is where he can expect to go when you return home if he misbehaves.

4. Take along a ballpoint or felt-tip pen. Tell the child in front of the public place that if she misbehaves, you will place a hash mark on the back of her hand. The child will then serve a minimum sentence in time-out at home for each hash mark on the hand.

trip to evaluate how their child has behaved and whether she has earned anything for good behavior. Your child with ADHD cannot wait while you delay the consequences for her good behavior. So dispense praise, approval, and points or tokens frequently throughout the trip. Don't give your child a chance to misbehave by ignoring the good things she may be doing and reacting only to the bad things.

■ *Evaluate the situation at the end.* Once the situation is over, give the child additional feedback about how you thought things went. Ask the child how he thought it went as well. Then dispense some additional rewards if the situation went especially well. And remember the rule in Principle 7—act, don't yak: talk less, touch more, and reward often.

Public places are notorious spots for parents to be reactive rather than proactive. That's because you are there for a reason—you have some goals to accomplish, errands to run, work to do, or even people to meet. But you can use this transition plan anytime, anywhere, when your child is transitioning from one major type of activity to another or from one setting to another. Let's say your family is going to visit your brother and his family, and you know your son with ADHD loves playing with his cousins and won't want to leave. To facilitate a smooth exit and a less endless car ride home, create a transition plan that lays out the rules, making the rewards for getting into and behaving while in the car particularly enticing. You can do the same when you have to get your child away from his favorite video game or outdoor activity to go to the dentist or some other unfavored appointment. Just adjust the value of the rewards to the difficulty the child will have with the particular transition, but try to stick with a pretty consistent punishment for all failures to follow the rules to keep these situations from becoming too negative. The best strategy for reducing problems with a child with ADHD is to be proactive as often as you can and not just react to all the problems your child may be throwing your way. Of course there will be unexpected events you will just have to cope with on the fly and maybe resort to reactive parenting, but even then you may find a strategy you used proactively in an earlier situation can bail you out.

Being proactive can help you prevent a lot of undesirable behavior from your child with ADHD. But what about those emotional meltdowns that we tend to see in kids with ADHD more than other children?

> **THE PROBLEM:** Children with ADHD have trouble regulating their emotions—and it's not because they lack skills.

As explained in the Introduction, children with ADHD don't regulate their own emotions very well. They are more impulsive when it comes to showing raw emotions, less able to inhibit them, and less able to employ the strategies we all use to moderate our emotions so that our expression of them is better suited to the current situation, less likely to cause conflict with others, and more likely to help achieve our longer-term goals. What can a parent do about this deficiency? Some of what you read above can help: Anticipating situations where your child is likely to feel disappointment, anger, frustration, or even elation can help you head off a meltdown or keep an ecstatic whirling dervish from wreaking havoc by modifying the situation or avoiding it entirely. Implementing a transition plan can help too. But not always. You may be able to rein in disruptive behavior, but you won't necessarily be able to keep your child from feeling a strong emotion and letting it rip.

> **THE SOLUTION:** Learn how emotions work so you can proactively intervene before strong emotions take hold.

What little research has been done on this problem to date has not found much in the way of psychological treatment that can help improve this area of executive deficits. Social skills training in which children are taught methods of anger control were not found to generalize to the real world outside of the training group situation. Working with children with ADHD one on one to teach them strategies to calm themselves when emotionally riled up was not much of a success either. The reason may be the same problem described earlier and repeated throughout this book—ADHD is more of a problem with using what you know, not one of knowing what to do. The few studies done to date on boosting emotion regulation all focused on teaching new skills—what to do. They were not designed to address the real problem—performance, or doing what you know. So teaching children with ADHD emotional control skills such as anger management is not likely to help them *use* those control strategies when faced with an emotional provocation in a real-life situation.

So, is there anything you could at least try that might help with this problem? Fortunately, yes, but these strategies all come from an understanding of how our emotions are triggered and therefore where we might be able to intervene to help ourselves manage them. The strategies modify the environment or your child's thoughts about a potentially upsetting situation to reduce the likelihood that she will have a strong emotional reaction to it. This idea flows naturally from one discussed earlier—if the problem is one of performing what we know (not knowing what to do), then altering the point of performance can help children with ADHD show what they know and better control their emotions in a situation.

Let's begin with how our emotions get triggered. In any given situation, we pay attention to what's going on, we appraise the situation, and we respond:

Situation → Attention → Appraisal → Response

Let's say your child with ADHD is at the playground and another child tries to take away the toy he is playing with or cut in front of him to take over the equipment he wanted to play on. Or maybe the other child says something teasing or even insulting to your son. But a potential emotionally triggering event has now occurred. For you, a triggering situation might be another driver suddenly cutting in front of you on the highway.

Once the child's emotional equilibrium is thrown off, this event gets his full, undivided attention, often very quickly and maybe exclusively. He stops paying attention to the larger context and focuses on the triggering event. You can see this in your child with ADHD when he turns his head quickly toward the provocation, his eyes widen, his mouth may drop open, and there is clearly a sign of unwelcome surprise on his face. This reaction of orienting to the trigger and focusing fully on it is almost reflexive, but not quite. If you were cut off by a rude, dangerous driver, you might suddenly be focusing all your attention on him and not on the road and the rest of the drivers. Your heart might be pounding as you imagine what could have happened if the driver had cut in just a few feet closer to your car.

Now the brain, often very quickly, evaluates this triggering event as a threat—something to be attacked (anger) or avoided (fear), fought or fled. For your child, this could just be a specific and discrete event, like someone taking a toy away from them during playtime at school or in your yard that quickly leads to frustration and even reactive aggression. But it might also be some protracted event that heightens his arousal and alertness more generally, such as a noisy birthday party where everyone is talking loudly, laughing, or having fun, so that over time it excites your child.

No matter what it is, the brain has quickly evaluated or appraised this triggering event as something that requires an emotional response. And so a response comes out—in the case of your child or teen with ADHD, often quickly (impulsively) and more strongly than might be seen in others. Sometimes this entire four-step sequence can occur within seconds, even semiconsciously, and it can feel like it is automatic and reflexive—something we can do nothing about with our conscious mind. And if a child has ADHD, once that emotion is triggered, it overwhelms the weak executive part of the brain, or the capacity for rational thinking, and so no amount of measured reasoning with a child at this point is going to do much good. The emotion just has to run its course before the executive brain can recover any modicum of even-temperedness and equilibrium.

Fortunately for all of us, it's not true that all this is simply automatic. Despite how fast this sequence occurs, seeing it as unfolding in four steps helps us see where we might intervene to change the likelihood of that emotional response.

The diagram below shows where and how you could change the course of an event and the emotions it triggers in the future. One caveat, though: *Research shows that the earlier in the sequence you make those changes, the more likely they are to succeed in preventing the triggered emotion or managing*

Six Places to Head Off Emotion Dysregulation

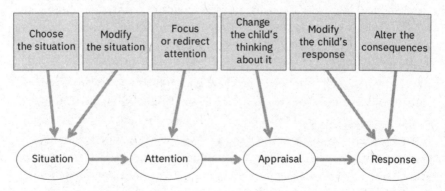

This diagram is based on descriptions of James J. Gross's modal model of emotion found in works published by Gross and his colleagues between 1998 and 2011.

it when it arises. In fact, trying to intervene later in the sequence may be effective only with older children, teens, and adults, who have had the time to develop their emotional self-regulation ability to some extent.

Choosing the Situation

Just as you did above in considering where your child is likely to behave inappropriately, look at those situations, places, or events that are most likely to trigger strong emotions in your child. Now select alternative situations to replace those. If the bully who sets your child off is likely to be at the playground on a certain day at a certain time, then for heaven's sake stop going to that playground at that time. Head off emotional problems by identifying emotionally provocative settings, events, or even people and then avoid them! Just as you might avoid taking your child with ADHD to a crowded supermarket on the way home from school because he's going to be hungry and restless and start grabbing candy and other snacks off the shelf, think about whether your child's greatest emotional difficulty is, say, frustration and avoid letting him play ball with his older, more athletic brother when the child with ADHD is already tired. There is no strong emotion that needs to be self-regulated if it is never provoked or triggered to begin with.

I know what you're thinking: How is my child supposed to learn emotional control and face such provocative situations unfazed if we simply avoid those situations and don't teach him the skills he needs to cope with them? Again, teaching skills here won't work because your child still won't use them in those situations where they would have helped. Second, for a child with a biological deficit in emotional self-control, this is a lot like saying to someone in a wheelchair who uses a ramp to enter a building, "How are you supposed to learn to enter that building using the stairs like the rest of us when you keep avoiding the steps and relying on that ramp?" Sounds pretty ridiculous when you put it that way, doesn't it? Biologically based problems are unlikely to just go away because we've taught the person skills intended to show her how to do something better. Instead, avoid exposing your child to a triggering event when you can. You won't have to do this forever, but for now keep doing it until more brain development occurs and your child's executive abilities progress to give her a little more emotional control.

Modifying the Situation

OK, you find yourself and your child in a situation you cannot avoid that could lead to an emotionally triggering event. What to do? Think about ways to modify that situation to reduce the chance that the emotional triggers will occur. Let's say you couldn't avoid the playground—your child's friends wanted to go there, or the bully showed up at a time or on a day when he's not usually there. In that case, move to the other side of the playground, where that bully tends not to play, or just turn around and walk out of the playground if you possibly can. Maybe you could invite the kids to play in your yard or home instead. Or let's say your son starts a game of catch with his older brother before you know what's happening, and you can already see the competition brewing and your child with ADHD getting frustrated and angry. Can you take your older son aside and ask him to take it easy on his little brother? Can you play with them and run interference? Can you set a time limit on the game and then suggest a game that the younger son can win (or at least compete at)? You've undoubtedly noticed that the "situation" includes not just the place, but the time and time period, the people involved, and exactly what's happening, so you might be able to make these modifications:

- *Modify the location.* Move to the other side of the playground, find a quieter spot for your child to play or study, or just leave the scene.

- *Modify the time or time period.* Exit the scene with the promise of returning when you know the trigger won't be present—the bully and other kids will have gone home, it won't be so hot outdoors, etcetera. Or cut things short. Put time limits on an activity that typically builds your child's frustration. Break things up into increments of activity with breaks in between.

- *Make modifications that involve the people on the scene.* Enlist the older brother's sympathetic help (with a reward as an incentive), steer your child toward an activity with one or two other children instead of a whole pack, help your child play with children who have the same EA if that's possible without bruising his pride, get other adults involved in the activity to keep things calm. I probably don't have to tell you not to invite the neighbor who always whips your child up to come play when your child is already on his last legs.

Focusing or Redirecting Your Child's Attention

We've all used this strategy from time to time. We are in a situation, and an emotionally provocative event has occurred. Now what? We stop looking at it, listening to it, or otherwise focusing on it. Maybe you look away, close your eyes, cover your eyes, turn around—do something to turn your attention from this event. There is a chance it may prevent the emotional reaction, but even if it doesn't it will help quell the intensity of your emotions and maybe even help you recover from them faster. Remember covering your ears or closing your eyes to avoid the scariest part of a horror movie?

So when you think about recurring situations that cause your child to become emotional, how could you shift your child's attention away from the provocative or triggering event? If your child is getting antsy while you're in the car or shopping and patient waiting often leads to a meltdown, protest, or tantrum, divert her attention from the act of waiting. Do you have something with you that your child can play with? Some paper to draw on? A game app on your smartphone she can play? Ringtones on your phone that she can cycle through and pick a new one? Maybe place a call to your partner so your child can speak with Mom or Dad while you wait? How about using that camera on the phone to let your child play photographer and shoot shots of whatever she wants? Modifying what a child is attending to is a third way of preventing or helping your child cope with emotionally provocative situations. The distractions listed earlier in the chapter under transition plans can be used to forestall inappropriately expressed emotions as well as heading off misbehavior.

Thinking ahead about what you could do to distract or modify your child's attention will pay dividends in the future because a meltdown can be upon you before you know it. If you are already in the situation, you'll have to think on your feet to come up with a distraction, so it's best to have some stored in your memory. If you find yourself in a checkout line with a 4-year-old who's about to explode at your "No" to candy, can you play peekaboo with your young child so she has to cover her eyes while you check out? Can you play a game of pulling your little boy's ski cap down over his eyes for laughs? Can you get the child to talk to the clerk or person in line ahead of you so his attention is diverted? Or better yet, before the tantrum even starts, quickly reach over, take a small candy package, open it, and tell your child she deserves this reward because she was so good while shopping with you today. Bingo, no meltdown.

Changing the Way Your Child Thinks about the Situation

I don't recommend you try this with young children with ADHD because it involves talking to them about the triggering event, why it is making them upset, reasons it is not as bad as they make it out to be, and other ways to think about what happened that help them cope with the strong emotion. You are teaching a form of reasoning here that requires reevaluating the significance of our thoughts and the events that triggered the emotion. Children with ADHD simply are not good at this because of all their executive function problems, including verbal self-speech. But with an older child or teen, questioning, reasoning, and even modeling what they can say to themselves to reduce the significance of the triggering event might work. Even then, however, the results of research on this approach are not very promising. This is cognitive-behavioral therapy, or CBT, and it is often used with adults or even children with anxiety or depression, for whom it works better. But it doesn't seem to work as well for people with ADHD until they reach adulthood. Yes, how we think about an event largely determines the emotions it triggers, but that's a pretty deep thought for a 6-year-old to understand when she is in the middle of an angry outburst, crying episode, or other display of strong emotion.

Modifying the Emotional Response

Of all the places to intervene to manage a strong emotion, this one is the least likely to succeed. I mention it here because it is part of the sequence of an emotion and some people, primarily adults, might be able to quell strong emotions, say by gritting their teeth, grabbing the sides of a table or chair they are sitting in, and just using good old willpower to try to inhibit the expression of the emotion, or at least acting on it. You can still see the emotion playing out on their face, but they are trying hard not to act it out physically in any other ways. I do not believe this is something that has any chance of working with a child or teen with ADHD, who is already suffering an impulse control problem.

However, there is another way you can implement this strategy—get your child an FDA-approved ADHD medication. Research shows that such medications don't just improve attention and inhibition; they improve the executive functions, including emotion dysregulation. Not always or for every child, but they may help with the majority of individuals who take these medications. So, here is another option in your toolkit to help you better manage your child's emotions. Consider ADHD medication.

Modifying the Consequences for the Emotion

This approach is simply using good old behavior modification methods—implementing negative consequences for misbehavior so it doesn't happen again while also providing reinforcement for episodes of emotional control that went well. It won't necessarily change the current emotional outburst. But it does have a small chance of changing the likelihood that it will happen again. In the various principles set forth here, I have covered many such strategies of using rewards and discipline to make the child or teen with ADHD more accountable for his behavior, and that can certainly include acting on emotions. So look for ways you can reward emotional control when your child handles a potential triggering event well and consider using response cost, fines, or time-out for excessive negative emotions out of proportion to the triggering event. Then be patient: it can take time for this type of training to succeed in improving your child's emotional control. However, it is unlikely to completely eliminate what is a largely biologically based problem with emotional self-regulation.

CONCLUSION

Putting It All Together

In this book I have set forth what I consider the 12 most important principles that you need to raise your child with ADHD. These principles are based on my work with thousands of families, numerous research studies I've conducted with those families, and more than four decades of following the research and personally working in the field of ADHD more generally. The Introduction to this book gave you a good foundation for understanding ADHD, and for more complete details you can turn to *Taking Charge of ADHD,* now in its fourth edition. In this book my goal has been to give you a helpful mindset and a toolbox full of strategies to help you cope with and manage your child's disorder but also—and just as important—to cultivate and maintain a good relationship with your child so that your child thrives, conflict is minimized, and your family functions smoothly and happily. The parents I've known have found that adopting these principles promotes the developmental, adaptive, and social effectiveness of their child while nurturing a close and supportive parent–child relationship.

You may not need all 12 principles or all of the specific methods discussed for addressing the deficits associated with them. If you've met a child with ADHD, then you have met only one child with ADHD. Your child is unique, and you know your son or daughter best. I hope you'll turn to the individual principles over and over as your child grows and find what you need when you need it—including reminders and support.

One way to remind yourself of the 12 principles is to photocopy the list below (or download and print it; see the end of the table of contents for more information) and place it where you'll see it every day—on your bathroom mirror, the refrigerator door, or the inside of your bedroom closet door, for example.

Besides the understanding of ADHD provided in the Introduction, I've found over 40 years that an important part of the foundation for raising a child with ADHD to thrive now and as an adult is forgiveness. As explained in Principle 2, it's important always to remember that your child has a disorder. Your son or daughter can't help behaving in atypical ways and sometimes being disruptive. With the 12 principles in mind, you can minimize that disruption, protect your child, and promote the child's adaptability and success. But there will be times when you will have to practice forgiveness—with your child, with yourself, and maybe even with those in your child's world who don't understand ADHD.

12 Principles for Raising a Child with ADHD

Principle 1. Use the Keys to Success

Principle 2. Remember That It's a Disorder!

Principle 3. Be a Shepherd, Not an Engineer

Principle 4. Get Your Priorities Straight

Principle 5. Mindful Parenting: Be There and Be Aware

Principle 6. Promote Your Child's Self-Awareness and Accountability

Principle 7. Touch More, Reward More, and Talk Less

Principle 8. Make Time Real

Principle 9. Working Memory Isn't Working: Offload It and Make It Physical!

Principle 10. Get Organized

Principle 11. Make Problem Solving Concrete

Principle 12. Be Proactive: Plan for Difficult Situations at Home and Away

From *12 Principles for Raising a Child with ADHD* by Russell A. Barkley. Copyright © 2021 The Guilford Press.

PRACTICE FORGIVENESS

As the parent of a child with a neurodevelopmental disorder of self-regulation, you are going to experience a far greater level of parenting stress than parents of typical children. That is because your child will need much more structure, supervision, and behavior management than other children. Being a parent of a child with ADHD seems like a 24/7 job. You may feel as if you always have to be on high alert for things that might go wrong due to your child's poorly regulated behavior. Your child is certainly not intentionally antagonizing you or making your life so distressing, but it can sometimes feel that way. Maybe it will help to remember what a special education teacher once told me: the children who need our love the most are likely to show it in the most unlikely ways. Your knowledge that your child has a brain-based problem with the capacity to self-regulate and the executive functions needed to do so should elicit empathy and compassion, as well as a willingness to make appropriate accommodations and to seek out the most effective evidence-based treatments.

But if that disability perspective sometimes isn't enough, one powerful way to help you alter your mindset and forgive your child is to rephrase the 12 principles as if your child with ADHD is asking you—even pleading with you—to follow them. The box on pages 178–179 shows what that might sound like.

If imagining your child imploring you to do these things didn't bring a tear to your eye, put a lump in your throat, and help you be a more understanding, compassionate, and forgiving parent, you'd probably be devoid of empathy toward your child. That seems highly unlikely. So with these pleas in mind, please give the principles serious consideration when raising your child or teen with ADHD. You won't regret it.

Forgiving Your Child

You also won't regret getting very good at forgiving your child. Having ADHD means making a lot more mistakes than other children. You know your child doesn't mean to behave this way. It is not some willful choice. Being 30% younger in EA means acting like someone 30% younger when it comes to self-control.

Forgiving your child for the mistakes he made due to that difference doesn't mean you don't try to help him behave better. You do that by using

An Open Letter from Your Child or Teen

Dear Mom and Dad: I really need your help and understanding of my ADHD.

1. I know I can succeed—but will need your love, support, and extra help to do so.

2. I didn't choose to be this way—but I need you to accept me for who I am.

3. My ADHD doesn't define everything about me—I have many unique strengths and aptitudes, and I'm your one-of-a-kind child—but I need you to protect me and create an environment where I can thrive.

4. I can't always do everything you want me to do, and I don't want to fight over it—so please let go of some things that don't matter so much to either of us and focus on the ones that do.

5. I can't control my behavior as well as other kids—but I really need you to notice when I'm being good so I'll remember how to behave better, and sometimes I just want to be with you and be appreciated.

6. I am not always aware that I am doing something wrong—help me become more aware of and monitor myself.

7. I can't motivate myself to work like other kids—you can help me stick with my work and get it done by giving me more external consequences, feedback, and accountability (and less yelling and talking).

8. Mom and Dad, I am "blind to time"—so try to be patient about that; help me cope with this by making time real (physical) and breaking down big projects into small steps with me.

9. I know I'm forgetful—there are things you can do to help me remember what I'm supposed to be doing.

10. OK, so I am not very organized—I can do that better if you teach me how to organize myself and my things.

11. I can't solve problems in my mind as well as others—help me get the pieces of the problem in my hands so I can solve it better.

12. Being away from home and my routines can make it even harder for me to focus and remember what to do—can you plan for trips to the store and other places so I can manage all the distractions and temptations and my emotions?

I Can't Handle My ADHD Alone— Please Let's Do This Together

the principles in this book. But it does mean that once you have a plan to help your child improve his behavior, you let go of all the emotions the latest mistake may have triggered and focus instead on how he can do this thing better the next time around. With your child, figure out what your plan is going to be to deal with that problem next time. Then let the last time go. Once your child understands that what he may have done was incorrect, and once you encourage him to apologize and make amends for any damages his mistake may have caused, focus on teaching him what to do instead. With that, end it—forgive.

This approach will benefit not only your child but also you. Having to intervene with your child as frequently as parents of kids with ADHD often do causes a lot of stress. The cumulative stress of these frequent daily interventions can result in irritability, anger, and resentment. There are many ways to cope with this stress, such as frequent exercise, yoga, meditation, arranging for "me time" or alone time more often, sharing parental responsibilities with your partner, or finding ways to rejuvenate yourself such as hobbies, friends, or a church group. Mindfulness, introduced in Principle 5, can be particularly helpful in learning to let go of distress. Self-care methods are discussed at more length in the fourth edition of *Taking Charge of ADHD*. Yet a surefire way to manage parental anger and distress is to forgive the child who seems to generate it.

So remind yourself often of your child's disability. Strive to approach her difficult behavior with compassion and constructive strategies. Find the irony and even humor in her misbehavior if you can. Then once she is back to behaving reasonably well, tell her you forgive her if that seems appropriate. At the very least, do so in your own mind.

And remember, as Paula Lawes wrote at *LifeHack.org,* forgiveness is not a gift you grant to others as much as it is a gift you give to yourself.

Forgiveness is not about letting the other person off the hook so easily or giving a gift you may not feel the other person deserves. It is a means of dispersing the mentally poisonous toxins that can accumulate in your mind from anger, hurt, grief, resentment, humiliation, and just plain old stress that has come your way from your interactions with another person—in this case your child or teen with ADHD.

A few parents over the many years of my clinical practice have taught me some things that they have found help them stay balanced emotionally, reduce stress, forgive their child with ADHD, and strive to be more loving and compassionate parents. I thought these coping methods were so useful that I have subsequently passed them on to other parents, and now on to you.

Put a picture of your child being good on the refrigerator door. One mother told me that she accidentally stumbled on this strategy, which really helped her remain relatively calm when dealing with the frequent misbehavior of her child with ADHD. One spring day he came in from playing outside with a handful of flowers he had picked from her flowerbed. He wanted her to have them as a gift. Rather than be angry about the destruction of her flower bed, she grabbed her smartphone, took a picture, printed it out, and put it on her refrigerator. There it serves as a daily reminder of who her child really is—a sweet, thoughtful, and kind child and not just a mischief maker. When she is upset with her son and losing control of her emotions, she goes to the refrigerator and looks long and hard at that picture. That is her real son, and not this momentarily evil twin that she has been grappling with that morning around various rule infractions and misbehaviors. It's a great idea to consider.

Have a daily exorcism! Another parent told me that the way he deals with his child's frequent misbehavior to reduce his stress levels is what he called the daily exorcism. At midday or the end of the day (or both!), he sits down with a sheet of paper and pencil and his favorite beverage for relaxation and makes a list of everything his daughter has done wrong so far that day. He even notes some of the more flagrant problems in capital letters with exclamation marks at the end. When he thinks he has made as complete a list as he can, and thus has fully vented his spleen over the confrontations with his daughter so far that day, he does something unusual. He steps outside onto their deck, takes a match, lights it, then sets fire to the lower corner of the paper and watches it slowly burn away. As it approaches his fingertips, he lets it go, and with it go all the hard feelings he may have been harboring toward his daughter that day. Then he utters, "I love you and I forgive you." Done, gone, exorcised from his mind and life. Maybe this strategy can work for you too.

Watch your child sleeping. This works better with younger children than teens, who might find what you are doing a tad creepy if they awaken. And a sleeping teen may not convey the image we seek here. One mother told me that when she has had a particularly bad day with her young child with ADHD, she finds a time after he has gone to bed and fallen asleep to tiptoe to his bedroom door, open it just enough to slide inside his room, and quietly find a place to sit on the floor with her back against a wall. Then she watches her child sleeping for a while. Few things convey a picture of innocence like a sleeping child. Melts your heart, doesn't it? How can you not let go of the hassles of the day while watching him sleep so innocently? And on really stressful days, she may even take a glass of chardonnay with her to sip while she tries to find peace with her child and herself in his room as he sleeps.

I am sure you have your own ways of finding private moments to reduce your stress, find some peace in your life, and let go of the stressful events of parenting that day. Maybe it's taking a bubble bath by candlelight with your favorite stress-reducing music on in the background. Or it's the opposite, such as going for a long run or for a workout at your health club while the kids are in bed and your partner is home to supervise them. Or it's a period of quiet contemplation and prayer or meditation in your favorite spot for such "me time." Or maybe you call a close friend with whom you can just talk through the day, or talk to your partner or spouse. At the end of them all comes that one magical act—forgiveness. Your child relies on you—for everything. You are the child's anchor, her rock, her guide, her therapist, teacher, protector, provider, and most of all, **you are your child's shepherd.**

Forgiving Yourself

The second reason you will need to practice forgiveness regarding your child with ADHD is to forgive yourself—often. Why? Because not only is your child going to make a lot of mistakes, but so will you. It comes with the role of being a parent. No one is a perfect parent; we *all* make mistakes in raising our children. The secret to raising well-adjusted children is not to avoid making any mistakes—that's impossible. It is to strive to get it right the next time that situation comes around again. It is to seek to be a better person as a result of mistake making. And the only way you can follow that advice is not to dwell on your mistakes, but to acknowledge that they happened, express apologies and regrets to the person you may have mistreated—and this definitely includes your child—and then let go of the mistake. You let go of the mistake with an act of self-forgiveness. You can say to yourself you now realize what you did or said wasn't right. You weren't the parent you want to be or know you can be. Promise yourself that you will try to do better next time and be a better parent for this child. Then let go of your distress by forgiving yourself for this mistake.

A Note about Forgiving Others

You know your child has a neurogenetic developmental disorder; others probably do not. You know your child therefore cannot always help behaving in atypical and disruptive ways; others do not. And you know that your child needs more understanding, compassion, and hands-on care and management than do other children as a consequence of his disability; others do not. Many times, especially when you're out in public or even with your friends and members of your extended family, other people may misinterpret the nature of your child's disruptive behavior and especially its source. They will judge not only your child's misbehavior but also you and your parenting skills harshly.

You're not going to be able to change the minds of all of these people or society at large, no matter how good an advocate you become for children with ADHD. So there is just one thing left for you to do to salvage your own peace of mind—forgive them! No, that's not going to change them either. But it might at least reduce *your* stress.

When someone is glaring at you or your child or makes a nasty remark, it's likely to set off mental arguments with the person, even recriminations and thoughts of revenge. But those responses tend to simply whip up your outrage. So I suggest engaging in some mental recovery methods we often teach in CBT. Examine where this person's own critical reactions came from. It's almost always ignorance of ADHD. This person doesn't really understand what you're going through and especially what your child is going through. And that's the other person's fault, the other person's problem—and you don't have to make it yours. Then practice forgiveness. You certainly don't have to express it out loud. Just say to yourself, "I forgive you your ignorance of my child's disability. I forgive you for your unfounded condemnation of my child and me." Many parents have found this is the quickest way to let go of anger, regret, or even humiliation. Then move on. Disengage from the encounter. Move to another space with your child and then get to a better place mentally as well.

CONSIDERING MEDICATION WHEN THE 12 PRINCIPLES AREN'T ENOUGH

Sometimes even when parents follow the principles set forth in this book, it's not enough to completely or effectively reduce all of the symptoms and impairments a child with ADHD may be experiencing. After all, it is a neurodevelopmental disorder. That implies some permanence of this condition across development for the majority of children diagnosed in childhood. What if using these 12 principles is not enough? Well, if a disorder is largely of a biological origin (like diabetes or epilepsy), as is ADHD, then sometimes we have to consider adding biological therapies. If a child or teen's ADHD is so impairing, so likely to lead to harm or even early death or a shortened life expectancy, and using the principles set forth here still leaves the child at such tremendous risk, then isn't it right to treat the child with a biological agent approved for the management of ADHD? As a parent, that is for you to decide. If you think your child may need more help than he's getting right now, I strongly encourage you to inform yourself about ADHD medications, which have been studied thoroughly and are discussed in detail in books like Dr. Timothy Wilens's *Straight Talk about Psychiatric Medications for Kids* and my *Taking Charge of ADHD*. But I also understand that parents have misgivings about trying psychiatric medications for children, so I focus here on dispelling the myths I've heard from many parents over the years. You might also be interested in the poignant story of one parent who found ADHD medications life changing for her young son with ADHD. On the Scary Mommy website, Rita Templeton describes how her son reacted to a trial of medication: "For the first time in . . . well, maybe his entire life, Colin seemed truly relaxed. But not in a stoned, disconnected way; more like a relieved way. Like someone who has finally been unburdened from the baggage that has unfairly saddled them for so long." (See the Resources for a link to the full story.)

Myths about ADHD Medications

1. *ADHD isn't a real disorder, and so using medications to manage it is just wrong.* Thousands of scientific studies on ADHD should have dispensed with this argument, but it still comes up. Real disorders are deficiencies in biologically based mental abilities that are universal in humans (everyone should develop them), and such deficiencies cause harm (greater mortality, morbidity, or impairment in major life activities). ADHD clearly meets these conditions, and so ADHD is a real disorder.

2. *ADHD may be a real disorder, but it's not the result of biological problems. It is the result of social factors, like diet, screen time, or poor upbringing. Therefore, medications are unwarranted as they just mask the real source of the problem.* ADHD *is* a biologically based disorder (see the fourth edition of *Taking Charge of ADHD* for more information), and therefore using biological agents like medications to help address it is warranted when psychological therapies are not enough to address it.

3. *ADHD medications are powerful, mind-altering drugs that can cause brain damage.* There is no evidence in the hundreds of neuroimaging or other studies to show that ADHD medications when taken as prescribed have any damaging influence on the child's brain or its development. Yes, if these drugs are abused in high doses and introduced into the body by other means, such as injection or inhalation, over extended periods some alterations to and damage of the brain can occur. But that is not how these medications are used for ADHD, so that is why no evidence of damage or impaired development has been found. Instead, there now exist at least 33 studies showing that extended treatment with ADHD stimulant medications may actually promote brain development in the regions of the brain associated with ADHD, which are often smaller than the same regions in typical brains.

4. *ADHD medications can lead to future risk for addiction to other drugs, especially other stimulants.* There are now more than 18 studies, including my own longitudinal study, that have found no evidence that treating children or teens with ADHD medications increases their risk for later drug use disorders. In fact, a few studies found that continuing to take

ADHD medications during adolescence reduced the future risk for certain types of drug use. Understand that children and teens with ADHD who have not been treated with ADHD medications have a significantly higher risk for later drug use disorders. It is therefore ADHD, and not the ADHD medications, that increases the later risk for addictions or other substance use problems. Treating ADHD should reduce those risks.

5. *It is best to try nonprescription alternative or natural therapies before trying a prescription ADHD medication.* I wish this were true. Studies show that many parents (more than 60%) have tried alternative or natural therapies for their child's ADHD before even discussing ADHD with their family physician. Such therapies, if effective, would offer us an easy and cheaper alternative to using prescription ADHD medications. But there are no natural, herbal, alternative, or other forms of therapy that are as effective for managing ADHD, and for as many people, as the FDA-approved ADHD medications.

6. *I should try psychological treatments with my child before considering medication for my child's ADHD.* This is not actually a myth. It's certainly what the Centers for Disease Control and Prevention, the American Academy of Pediatrics, and other organizations have recommended. And for a child with mild ADHD who is not in urgent need of treatment, this may make some sense. But for moderate to severe ADHD or where harm may be imminent for the child or teen if the disorder is left untreated for long, such an approach does not make sense. Psychological treatments can take a lot longer to produce benefits than can medications, they produce less improvement than medication, and they require consistent implementation from an adult that may not be possible in all settings (such as while a teen is driving).

COMING FULL CIRCLE: CHANGING YOUR MINDSET TO CHANGE HOW YOU UNDERSTAND AND CARE FOR YOUR CHILD WITH ADHD

The principles in this book are designed to help you reach the goals I set out at the beginning: to understand ADHD and use the keys to success that I've identified as instrumental in raising a happy, healthy child with ADHD (see Principle 1). The first few principles focus on changing your mindset about ADHD and your child. I wanted you to understand

ADHD as many other clinical scientists and I have come to understand it—as a neurodevelopmental disorder of the executive functions and the self-regulation they permit. The fact that your child, due to no fault of her own, is far less able than other children to control her own behavior is the reason you've had to intervene much more than parents of typical children to help manage the child, protect her from harm, and nurture her development. If you have come to understand ADHD this way, several of my other aims in writing this book may have been achieved.

One of those is to foster acceptance of your child for who she is, not what you wanted her to be. It was to instill the perspective that you are a shepherd, not an engineer. You cannot design your children, and you cannot redesign them to get rid of their ADHD. Another aim was to promote a more mindful approach to parenting so that you can better attend to, evaluate, reward, and otherwise support your child and help her become better adjusted. I also hoped that through a better, deeper understanding of ADHD and the concept of being a mindful shepherd to your child or teen you would also develop a sense of compassion and forgiveness toward your child. If you've read and started applying the dozen principles in this book, you have likely developed a more accurate, more helpful, and less stressful frame of mind for raising your child with ADHD.

Our mental frames of reference are powerful influences in our lives because they organize our understanding of life and in this case of our children. In so doing they largely determine the kinds of decisions we make and actions we take in meeting the demands of life and in raising our children. With your new perspective on your child's ADHD, you are now in a better position to put in place the kinds of accommodations you need to make so that your child is less disabled by ADHD. In other words, the strategies that flow from the 12 principles can help your child adapt, function, and succeed. They also help you toward modifying your own behavior so that you can be a more effective and loving parent. And, in turn, they give you ways to help modify your child's behavior so that he can be more successful in what he must do while maintaining a close relationship with you.

MY WISH FOR YOU

I wish you all success in applying these basic principles with your child or teen with ADHD. I hope that you find them to be of value to you for better managing your child or teen with ADHD. There is no higher compliment a clinician and clinical researcher can receive than to learn that parents like you have benefited from my life's work in this field. These principles come from that life's work. It is also my wish for you that in using these principles, you have not only reduced your child's ADHD and related impairments, but more importantly, that you have greatly improved and strengthened the relationship you have with your child. That relationship can sustain you both throughout your life.

RESOURCES

Many sources of additional information, support, and advice are available on the Internet for parents of children with ADHD. The following list is divided up by the principles in this book.

PRINCIPLE 1. USE THE KEYS TO SUCCESS

ADDitude magazine:
   www.additudemag.com/adhd-success-stories-6-superstars-with-attention-deficit
   www.additudemag.com/adhd-success-stories-teacher
   www.additudemag.com/slideshows/famous-people-with-adhd
Beyond Book Smart: *www.beyondbooksmart.com/executive-functioning-strategies-blog/overcoming-the-challenges-of-adhd*
Child Mind Institute: *https://childmind.org/blog/adam-levine-speaks-out-about-his-adhd*
Healthline: *www.additudemag.com/slideshows/famous-people-with-adhd*
Understood: *www.understood.org/en/learning-thinking-differences/child-learning-disabilities/add-adhd/adhd-success-stories*

PRINCIPLE 2. REMEMBER THAT IT'S A DISORDER!

Attention Deficit Disorders Association: *www.add.org*
Centre for ADHD Awareness, Canada: *www.caddac.ca*
Child Mind Institute: *www.childmind.org*
Children and Adults with ADHD: *www.chadd.org*
Help for ADHD: *www.help4adhd.org*
Russell A. Barkley, PhD (Fact Sheets): *russellbarkley.org*
World Federation for ADHD: *www.adhd-federation.org*

PRINCIPLE 3. BE A SHEPHERD, NOT AN ENGINEER

Scientific American: www.scientificamerican.com/article/parents-peers-children
Very Well Mind: *www.verywellmind.com/what-is-nature-versus-nurture-2795392*

Books

Pinker, S. (2002). *The blank slate.* New York: Penguin.
Rich Harris, J. (2009). *The nurture assumption.* New York: Free Press.

PRINCIPLE 4. GET YOUR PRIORITIES STRAIGHT

Families.com: *www.families.com/what-should-a-good-parents-priorities-be*
KidsHealth: *https://kidshealth.org/en/parents/nine-steps.html*
Parent Circle: *www.parentcircle.com/article/5-priorities-for-good-parenting/*
Parenting the Modern Family: *www.parentingthemodernfamily.com/rule-2-be-a-purposeful-parent-parent-with-priorities*
Parenting: The Biggest Job: *www.biggestjob.com/about/the-10-priorities*

PRINCIPLE 5. MINDFUL PARENTING:
BE THERE AND BE AWARE

Aha! Parenting: *www.ahaparenting.com/parenting-tools/peaceful-parenting/mindful-parenting*
Child Mind Institute: *https://childmind.org/article/mindful-parenting-2*
Goop.com: *https://goop.com/work/parenthood/the-four-keys-to-mindful-parenting*
Gottman Institute: *www.gottman.com/blog/mindful-parenting-how-to-respond-instead-of-react*
Greater Good Magazine: *https://greatergood.berkeley.edu/article/item/mindful_parenting_may_keep_kids_out_of_trouble*
Huffington Post: *www.huffpost.com/entry/the-5-main-tenets-of-mindful-parenting_n_4086080*
Mind Body Green: *www.mindbodygreen.com/0-29429/9-mindful-parenting-tips-for-when-youre-about-to-lose-your-cool.html*
Mindful: Healthy Mind, Healthy Life: *www.mindful.org/5-mindful-tips-for-parenting-conundrums*
PsychAlive: *www.psychalive.org/benefits-of-mindful-parenting*
Washington Post: www.washingtonpost.com/news/parenting/wp/2014/08/26/how-i-learned-to-be-a-more-mindful-parent/?noredirect=on

Books

Bertin, M. (2015). *Mindful parenting of ADHD*. Oakland, CA: New Harbinger.

Kabat-Zinn, J. (2005). *Wherever you go, there you are*. New York: Hachette Books.

Kabat-Zinn, J., & Kabat-Zinn, M. (1998). *Everyday blessings: The inner work of mindful parenting*. New York: Hachette Books.

Race, K. (2014). *Mindful parenting: Simple and powerful solutions for raising creative, engaged, happy kids in today's hectic world*. Spokane, WA: St. Martin's Griffin.

PRINCIPLE 6. PROMOTE YOUR CHILD'S SELF-AWARENESS AND ACCOUNTABILITY

Self-Awareness

Exploring Your Mind: *https://exploringyourmind.com/4-ways-promote-self-awareness-children*

Leaderonomics: *https://leaderonomics.com/personal/child-self-awareness*

Learning Works for Kids: *http://cdn2.hubspot.net/hub/287778/file-231442306-pdf/improving_self-awareness.pdf%3Cb%3E%3C/b%3E*

MomJunction: *www.momjunction.com/articles/teach-self-awareness-to-your-child_00359060/#gref*

Parent Tool Kit (tips for kindergarten age children): *www.parenttoolkit.com/social-and-emotional-development/advice/self-awareness/kindergarten-self-awareness-tips*

Psychology Today: *www.psychologytoday.com/us/blog/the-moment-youth/201508/self-awareness-how-kids-make-sense-life-experiences*

Roots of Action: *www.rootsofaction.com/self-awareness-meaning-purpose*

Understood: *www.understood.org/en/friends-feelings/empowering-your-child/self-awareness/the-importance-of-self-awareness*

You Are Mom: *https://youaremom.com/education/self-awareness-children*

Accountability

Aha! Parenting: *www.ahaparenting.com/parenting-tools/character/responsibility*

Center for Parenting Education: *https://centerforparentingeducation.org/library-of-articles/responsibility-and-chores/developing-responsibility-in-your-children*

Empowering Parents: *www.empoweringparents.com/article/how-to-create-a-culture-of-accountability-in-your-home*

A Fine Parent: *https://afineparent.com/building-character/personal-accountability.html*

Books

Barkley, R. A., & Benton, C. (2013). *Your defiant child: 10 steps to better behavior*. New York: Guilford Press.

Barkley, R. A., Robin, A. R., & Benton, C. (2013). *Your defiant teen*. New York: Guilford Press.

Bertin, M. (2011). *The family ADHD solution*. Spokane, WA: Griffin.

PRINCIPLE 7. TOUCH MORE, REWARD MORE, AND TALK LESS

American Psychological Association (parenting tips): *www.apa.org/helpcenter/communication-parents*

Child Development Institute (20 Ways to Talk So Your Kids Will Listen): *https://childdevelopmentinfo.com/how-to-be-a-parent/communication/talk-to-kids-listen*

Parents.com: *www.parents.com/parenting*

Peaceful Parent: *https://peacefulparent.com/peaceful-parenting-basic-principles*

Psychology Today: *www.psychologytoday.com/us/basics/parenting* and *www.psychologytoday.com/us/blog/the-mindful-self-express/201209/worst-mistakes-parents-make-when-talking-kids*

Raising Children Network: *https://raisingchildren.net.au/toddlers/connecting-communicating/communicating/communicating-well-with-children*

Today's Parent: *www.todaysparent.com/family/age-by-age-guide-to-getting-your-kid-to-talk*

Very Well Family: *www.verywellfamily.com/how-do-you-talk-to-your-child-620058*

PRINCIPLE 8. MAKE TIME REAL

Great Schools: *www.greatschools.org/gk/articles/time-management-for-kids*

Scholastic.com: *www.scholastic.com/parents/family-life/parent-child/teach-kids-to-manage-time.html*

Timers: *www.timetimer.com*; *www.online-stopwatch.com/classroom-timers*; *www.lakeshorelearning.com/products/ca/p/EA165*

Very Well Family: *www.verywellfamily.com/how-to-teach-your-kids-time-management-skills-4126588*

PRINCIPLE 9. WORKING MEMORY ISN'T WORKING: OFFLOAD IT AND MAKE IT PHYSICAL!

ADDitude magazine: *www.additudemag.com/working-memory-exercises-for-children-with-adhd*

Charlotte Parent: *www.charlotteparent.com/CLT/Helping-Your-Forgetful-Child-Remember*

Developing Minds: *https://developingminds.net.au/blog/2016/11/15/fixes-for-forgetful-kids*

Family Matters: *www.ronitbaras.com/family-matters/parenting-family/how-to-cure-a-forgetful-kid*

Focus on the Family: *www.focusonthefamily.com/parenting/age-appropriate-chores*

MetroKids: *www.metrokids.com/MetroKids/January-2010/A-Forgetful-Child-Strategy*

Parenting: *https://parenting.firstcry.com/articles/15-ways-to-help-forgetful-kids-remember-stuff*

Positive Parenting: *https://positiveparenting.com/parenting-forgetful-behavior*

Scholastic: *www.scholastic.com/parents/books-and-reading/raise-a-reader-blog/what-to-do-when-your-child-cant-remember-what-he-reads.html*

Understood: *www.understood.org/en/school-learning/learning-at-home/homework-study-skills/8-working-memory-boosters*

WatchMinder: *www.watchminder.com*

WebMD: *www.webmd.com/parenting/features/chores-for-children*

PRINCIPLE 10. GET ORGANIZED

Alejandra: *www.alejandra.tv/home-organizing-videos/kids-toys-back-to-school-organizing-ideas*

Clutterbug: *www.youtube.com/watch?v=AnQHLeK4cto*

Coolmompicks: *https://coolmompicks.com/blog/2017/09/12/creative-kids-workspace-ideas-how-to-make*

Good Housekeeping: *www.goodhousekeeping.com/home/organizing/tips/g340/organizing-tips-for-kids*

HGTV (recommendations for organizing broken down by age group): *www.hgtv.com/design/rooms/kid-rooms/get-your-kids-organized-at-all-ages*

House Beautiful: *www.housebeautiful.com/home-remodeling/g2270/10-genius-storage-ideas-for-your-kids-room*

KidsHealth.org: *https://kidshealth.org/en/parents/child-organized.html*

Organized Home: *www.organized-home.com/posts/childrens-rooms-workspace-roundup*

Parents: *www.parents.com/kids/education/back-to-school/how-to-create-homework-hq*

Scholastic: *www.scholastic.com/parents/school-success/homework-help/school-organization-tips/design-kid-friendly-workspace.html*

PRINCIPLE 11. MAKE PROBLEM SOLVING CONCRETE

All Pro Dad: *www.allprodad.com/10-ways-to-teach-your-children-to-be-problem-solvers*

Big Life Journal: *https://biglifejournal.com/blogs/blog/how-teach-problem-solving-strategies-kids-guide*

Bright Horizons (for young children): *www.brighthorizons.com/family-resources/developing-critical-thinking-skills-in-children*

Head Start Early Childhood Learning and Knowledge Center (a video webinar): *https://eclkc.ohs.acf.hhs.gov/teaching-practices/teacher-time-series/its-big-problem-teaching-children-problem-solving-skills*

Heart-Mind Online: *https://heartmindonline.org/resources/5-step-problem-solving-for-young-children*

Raising Children: *https://raisingchildren.net.au/grown-ups/looking-after-yourself/communication-conflict/problem-solving-for-parents*

Scholastic: *www.scholastic.com/teachers/articles/teaching-content/how-you-can-help-children-solve-problems*

Very Well Family: *www.verywellfamily.com/teach-kids-problem-solving-skills-1095015*

PRINCIPLE 12. BE PROACTIVE: PLAN FOR DIFFICULT SITUATIONS AT HOME AND AWAY

Childhood 101: *https://childhood101.com/parenting-styles-reactive-or-proactive*

Clear Expectations: *http://clear-expectations.net/being-a-proactive-parent*

Equinox Family Consulting: *https://equinoxfamilyconsulting.com/anxiety/proactive-or-reactive-which-would-you-rather-be*

The Family Room (Bright Horizons): *https://blogs.brighthorizons.com/familyroom/5-tips-for-positive-and-proactive-parenting*

MassPartnership.com: *www.masspartnership.com/pdf/ProactiveParenting.pdf*

Momables: *www.momables.com/becoming-a-proactive-parent-podcast*

Momtastic.com: *www.momtastic.com/parenting/701285-10-steps-becoming-proactive-parent-child-deserves*

Proactive Parenting: *https://proactiveparenting.net*

Racheous: *www.racheous.com/respectful-parenting/reactive-vs-proactive*

Scholarship Archives at Brigham Young University: *https://scholarsarchive.byu.edu/cgi/viewcontent.cgi?article=1415&context=marriageandfamilies*

CONCLUSION: PUTTING IT ALL TOGETHER

Catholic Exchange: *https://catholicexchange.com/five-ways-to-practice-forgiveness-2*

Dr. Wayne Dyer: *www.drwaynedyer.com/blog/how-to-forgive-someone-in-15-steps*

Forgiveness Practice (YouTube): *www.youtube.com/watch?v=I0UT7x8aX-A*

Greater Good in Action: *https://ggia.berkeley.edu/practice/nine_steps_to_forgiveness*

Huffington Post (Life Section): *www.huffpost.com/entry/forgiveness-tips_n_3306557*

Jack Kornfield (Buddhist teachings): *https://jackkornfield.com/the-practice-of-forgiveness*

Journey (New Life Christian Church): *http://journey.newchurch.org/programs/practicing-forgiveness*

LifeHack.org: *www.lifehack.org/articles/communication/how-practice-forgiveness-and-happier.html*

Mindful: *www.mindful.org/practice-self-compassion-with-forgiveness*

Safety and Health: *www.safetyandhealthmagazine.com/articles/14670-all-about-you-practicing-forgiveness*

Scary Mommy: *www.scarymommy.com/why-parenting-my-son-with-adhd-is-like-hugging-a-butterfly*

Spirituality and Health: *https://spiritualityhealth.com/articles/2018/09/20/the-power-of-practicing-forgiveness*

Strongest Families Institute: *www.strongestfamilies.com*

Tips on Life and Love: *www.tipsonlifeandlove.com/self-help/how-to-practice-forgiveness*

Writing Cooperative: *https://writingcooperative.com/why-practice-forgiveness-f1e24905c00e*

INDEX

Note. *f* following a page number indicates a figure.

ABOUT THE AUTHOR

Russell A. Barkley, PhD, ABPP, ABCN, before retiring in 2021, served on the faculties of the University of Massachusetts Medical Center, the Medical University of South Carolina, and Virginia Commonwealth University. Dr. Barkley has worked with children, adolescents, and families since the 1970s and is the author of numerous bestselling books for both professionals and the public, including *Taking Charge of ADHD* and *Your Defiant Child*. He has also published six assessment scales and more than 300 scientific articles and book chapters on attention-deficit/hyperactivity disorder, executive functioning, and childhood defiance. A frequent conference presenter and speaker who is widely cited in the national media, Dr. Barkley is past president of the Section on Clinical Child Psychology (the former Division 12) of the American Psychological Association (APA), and of the International Society for Research in Child and Adolescent Psychopathology. He is a recipient of awards from the American Academy of Pediatrics and the APA, among other honors. His website is *http://www.russellbarkley.org.*